The Nature of
Childhood Autism

The Nature of
Childhood Autism

SECOND EDITION

Gerald O'Gorman
F.R.C.P., D.P.M.

Physician Superintendent,
Borocourt Hospital, Reading,
Berkshire

LONDON: BUTTERWORTHS

ENGLAND:	BUTTERWORTH & CO. (PUBLISHERS) LTD. LONDON: 88 Kingsway, W.C.2B 6AB
AUSTRALIA:	BUTTERWORTH & CO. (AUSTRALIA) LTD. SYDNEY: 20 Loftus Street MELBOURNE: 343 Little Collins Street BRISBANE: 240 Queen Street
CANADA:	BUTTERWORTH & CO. (CANADA) LTD. TORONTO: 14 Curity Avenue, 374
NEW ZEALAND:	BUTTERWORTH & CO. (NEW ZEALAND) LTD. WELLINGTON: 49/51 Ballance Street AUCKLAND: 35 High Street
SOUTH AFRICA:	BUTTERWORTH & CO. (SOUTH AFRICA) LTD. DURBAN: 33/35 Beach Grove

©
Butterworth & Co. (Publishers) Ltd.
1970

Suggested U.D.C. Number: 616.89–053.2

ISBN 0 407 32601 4

Printed in Great Britain by
R. J. Acford Ltd.
Industrial Estate
Chichester
Sussex

Contents

Preface

Childhood autism is no longer thought to be excessively rare; but certainly it is still excessively difficult to understand. This is partly because the term is used with different meanings by different people; some regarding it as a 'disease' like pneumonia or cancer or encephalitis lethargica, others seeing it as a syndrome or collection of symptoms, while others again use the term autism as being equivalent to 'withdrawal' and denoting a process-symptom which is usually, but not necessarily associated with certain other symptoms to constitute the so-called 'autistic syndrome' or 'schizophrenic syndrome in childhood'. Autism is regarded by some as a symptom or as a complication of mental sub-normality. Some authorities regard it as an organic disease of the central nervous system; other believe it is predominantly a pattern of reaction to emotional stress. It is alleged to have close relationship with adult schizophrenia, with hysteria, and with other psychiatric illnesses. Autistic children are exceedingly difficult to treat or to educate; they arouse severe anxieties and emotional strain in their families and in those who care for them. Every aspect of childhood autism is at present a subject of acute controversy and the number of cases diagnosed increases all the time. It is, therefore, a condition of some importance medically, educationally and sociologically.

For these reasons it seemed advisable at this time to enquire into the true nature of childhood autism.

G. O'GORMAN

CHAPTER 1

WHAT IS CHILDHOOD AUTISM?

It would be convenient if one could give, in a few words, a precise definition of childhood autism and then proceed to describe its manifestations and course. This unfortunately is not possible in the present state of our knowledge. There is much debate and not a little confusion about the delineation of autism, mostly because nobody has yet been able to produce an acceptable analysis of the nature of the condition. Most children's psychiatrists would agree as to the diagnosis in the majority of cases. But there are a large number of children whom one psychiatrist would regard as autistic but whom others would not include in this group; and there are many individual symptoms which some would regard as manifestations of autism whilst others would disagree.

This book is an attempt to enquire into the essential nature of childhood autism. If a definition is to be achieved it can only come at the end of the book. However, the reader with no great experience of childhood autism needs to have some preliminary idea about the kind of child we are discussing; and perhaps this can best be afforded by describing two typical but contrasting cases.

Case No. 1. Mary. Admitted to Smiths Hospital aged four years

Mother's description—Ignores all of us; will not stay near the baby, uses me as a tool; will not play with toys; acts as though she is deaf.

History—Pregnancy and labour were normal. Mother was Rhesus negative but there was no neonatal jaundice. A lively baby, she fed normally at the breast for four months, and was weaned easily. All milestones were passed normally except that after

' mama ' and ' dada ' at six months there were no further words, apart from a few rare but appropriate phrases between two and three years. The only separation from mother was at 15 months when mother was in hospital for eight days for the birth of Mary's younger brother. Mary withdrew progressively from the age of about 12 months, when her mother was in the middle of her pregnancy with this next child, and increasingly after his birth. She became very agitated when mother handled the baby or put him in her pram, and she refused to be cuddled. She was aggressive to the baby and to herself. She developed head banging, a peculiar gait, a dreamy expression and inappropriate smiles. She became preoccupied with switches and surfaces and tongue sensations, and ceased to play or to make any relationship with other children. Mother brought her to the clinic at the age of two years eleven months. She was treated as an out-patient for one year without improvement.

Mental state—After admission she slowly became pot trained, learned to feed and dress herself. She became less withdrawn and made a real, though episodic, relationship with her mother (whom she saw weekly or more often) and with the nurses. However, she made hardly any contact with children. At the age of 5½ years she showed occasional and inconsistent squint, she indulged in strange mannerisms with her hands, she would not look at people or at things which people wanted her to look at, and she had occasional tantrums with wild monotonous screaming or moaning. Her gait was awkward and restless. She made only occasional responses to spoken words, although her hearing was evidently normal. She said a few phrases, unexpectedly but appropriately, but usually only made baby noises. There were no abnormal signs on examination of the central nervous system.

Treatment was aimed at promoting the mother–child relationship and getting Mary and the family to accept one another. Mother, though she tried, was never able to spare as much time for Mary as she needed because of the demands of her job and the rest of the family. Mary remained obviously jealous of the siblings, but mother found it hard even to visit her in the hospital without bringing the demanding younger brother with her. As the years went by the family were less, not more, able to tolerate Mary's

2

illness. She behaved well when taken home if alone in the house with mother. But as soon as anyone else came in she became very disturbed, screaming and smashing, taking off her clothes and wandering into neighbours' gardens. At the age of 12, with the onset of puberty, she became more violent, and there seemed to be an element of calculated cunning in the mischief and assaults she perpetrated. She had to be moved to the adult hospital where it was physically easier to contain her. Attempts at intensive occupation were continued, and she quietened a little. But she presented an absolutely typical picture of severe catatonic schizophrenia—manneristic, posturing and impulsively violent.

Case No. 2. Jonathan. Admitted to Smiths Hospital aged two years ten months

Mother's complaint—Plays in a peculiar way with his hands; frequently laughs inanely at nothing; screws up his eyes to look at lights; refuses to eat anything except biscuits; will not look at his parents or his brother; increasingly solitary.

History—Jonathan was regarded as normal up to 11 months. Milestones were passed at normal times but at 11 months his parents left him with a maternal grandmother whilst they went on holiday, during which time he screamed constantly day and night, was unresponsive to people and no longer played. He ignored his parents on their return. He had been saying a few words, like a normal baby of 11 months, but these he lost and he was not speaking at the time of admission to hospital. At 15 months his younger brother was born and his behaviour deteriorated further. He became increasingly manneristic and solitary. When first examined at the age of 2 years and 5 months, he was withdrawn, making no relationships with anyone. He showed many peculiar mannerisms, including looking at everything between his fingers, and facial grimaces. He had a variable squint, he did not play with toys, he would not look at people but seemed to 'look through' them, he at times showed no response to the spoken word although it was evident that he could hear well. He did not play with other children.

On admission to hospital he made no attempt to speak. He would go to anyone but made no emotional attachments. After about a

3

month he began to make relationships with the staff. At 3 years 6 months he was making good relationships with the staff and animals, but he did not as yet play with the other children. Speech began—as monosyllables—at 3 years 10 months, but he was saying no more words at the age of 4 years 3 months. In every other way he was making steady progress. He played normally with other children and with toys, and understood everything that was said to him. However, he was excessively timid and still had periods when he would withdraw completely, especially when exposed to strange people or a strange situation. At 5 years 3 months he was still speaking only in monosyllables, but his speech improved rapidly from the age of about 5¾. He was using an almost normal range of vocabulary for his age by the time he was 6½ though his articulation was still very faulty.

He had continued to see his family regularly whilst at Smiths, but the frequency of his visits was increased progressively as his condition improved and his tolerance of his younger siblings increased. After 3 years of intensive teaching in very small groups in the hospital school he left hospital and went to an ordinary primary school, in which he joined normally in the lessons and the play, though still rather timid and diffident about speaking. At the age of 7 years 7 months the psychologist reported, ' He now forms long complex sentences and uses nearly all parts of speech, including disjunctives, appropriately '.

At three years one month he had been untestable on ordinary intellectual tests, but on the Vineland Social Maturity Scale his social quotient was 56. At six years his mental age on the Merrill Palmer test was assessed at six years two months. At the age of seven years seven months his I.Q. on the Weschler Intelligence Scale for Children (W.I.S.C.) was: Verbal scale, 100; Performance scale, 101; Full scale I.Q., 101. His reading was six months retarded and his drawing one year retarded.

By his eighth birthday Jonathan was completely normal in every way both as regards his school work and his relationship with other children and adults. He was noted as having great poise and charm but as holding his own normally in arguments with other children. He was now in the A stream at his primary school.

CHILDHOOD PSYCHOSES

In the years immediately following World War II the attention of child psychiatrists was directed, to a much greater degree than previously, to what were called psychotic illnesses of childhood, or the childhood psychoses. No precise and generally accepted definition has emerged of what is meant by psychoses, but most psychiatrists were prepared to distinguish psychotic reactions in childhood from other types of mental disturbance. The criteria upon which this distinction was based often appeared to be nebulous, although the most experienced clinicians in this field generally agree about a particular case. Gradually, however, it became increasingly evident that ' psychosis ' is not a sufficient diagnosis by itself (Rimland, 1962). Indeed, it would not be surprising if there were as many different types of psychotic reaction in children as there are in adults. It is a fact of any psychiatrist's experience that the greater the number of adult patients seen, the smaller is the percentage that can be fitted exclusively and without reservation into any of the traditionally accepted diagnostic groups. In fact, there seems to be a tendency to think less of disease entities like ' hebephrenia ' or ' acute mania ', for example, except as a kind of shorthand for describing the most prominent features of the case, and to think more in terms of reaction types, recognizing that an individual patient may show features of two or even more of these types of reaction. For example, one may say that a patient is reacting in some ways schizophrenically, but that he is also depressed.

If we approach the patient with the idea of reaching a firm ' diagnosis '—as we do in a case of pneumonia for example—and of then ' curing ' him with drugs or injections or operations, we may have only limited success. We have to recognize that the patient must be helped to readjust himself to an environment in which he has already broken down. The psychiatrist has to think not of a person suffering from a

5

' disease ', but of one reacting to environmental circumstances with which, for the time being, he cannot cope because of the individual and particular nature of his hereditary constitution, his metabolism, his intelligence and his previous experience.

If the above is true of adults it is also presumably true of children. Nevertheless the psychiatrists, following the classical methods of general medicine, attempted to separate psychotic children into various clinical groups—' childhood schizophrenia ', ' the schizophrenic syndrome ', ' infantile autism ', ' Kanner's syndrome ', ' hyperkinetic syndrome ', ' Mahler's syndrome ', ' Heller's syndrome ', to mention only a few. It was not clear whether these were different names for the same condition, or different conditions having certain features in common. In fact, clinical experience seems to show that hardly any patients fitted exactly into the groups included under these names, and almost every new case of childhood psychosis seemed to have new and different features. The situation with regard to diagnosing and understanding childhood psychoses was therefore most confused.

THE SCHIZOPHRENIC SYNDROME—
' THE NINE POINTS '

In 1961, a Working Party convened by Dr. E. M. Creak (Creak, 1961) put forward certain criteria of diagnosis of what they called ' The Schizophrenic Syndrome in Childhood ' in an effort to delineate the syndrome and so have a basis for teaching and research on this subject. The working party used the term ' schizophrenic syndrome ' rather than ' schizophrenia ' because they felt that there was not sufficient evidence that this condition or ' reaction type ' they were describing was truly analogous to adult schizophrenia. The name ' childhood autism ' seemed at the time to be too narrow, for it seemed that autism described only a part of the syndrome. The term ' childhood psychosis ', on the other

6

hand, was rejected as being too wide, including as it must such conditions as depression and disturbances due to head injury or to toxic or infective states.

The working party eventually put forward criteria for diagnosis of the schizophrenic syndrome in childhood, without in any way committing themselves as to the nature of the syndrome or its aetiology. The criteria in their revised form are as follows:

(1) Gross and sustained impairment of emotional relationships with people; this includes the more usual aloofness and empty clinging (so-called symbiosis), also abnormal behaviour towards other people as persons, such as using them or parts of them impersonally; difficulty in mixing and playing with other children is often outstanding and long lasting.

(2) Apparent unawareness of the child's own personal identity to a degree inappropriate to his age; this may be seen in abnormal behaviour towards himself, such as posturing or exploration and scrutiny of parts of his body; repeated self-directed aggression, sometimes resulting in actual damage, may be another aspect of his lack of integration (*see also* (5)), also the confusion of personal pronouns (*see* (7)).

(3) Pathological preoccupation with particular objects or certain characteristics of them, without regard to their accepted functions.

(4) Sustained resistance to change in the environment and a striving to maintain or restore sameness; in some instances behaviour appears to aim at producing a state of perceptual monotony.

(5) Abnormal perceptual experience (in the absence of discernible organic abnormality), implied by excessive, diminished or unpredictable response to sensory stimuli, for example, visual and auditory avoidance—*see also* (2) and (4) —or insensitivity to pain or temperature.

(6) Acute, excessive and seemingly illogical anxiety. This is a frequent phenomenon and tends to be precipitated by

change, whether in material environment or in routine, as well as by temporary interruption of a symbiotic attachment to persons or things—compare (3) and (4) and also (1) and (2). Apparently commonplace phenomena or objects seem to become invested with terrifying qualities. On the other hand, an appropriate sense of fear in the face of real danger may be lacking.

(7) Speech may have been lost, or never acquired, or may have failed to develop beyond a level appropriate to an earlier stage. There may be confusion of personal pronouns—*see* (2)—echolalia or other mannerisms of use or diction. Although words or phrases may be uttered, they may convey no sense of ordinary communication.

(8) Distortion in motility patterns, for example, excess as in hyperkinesis, immobility as in katatonia, bizarre postures or ritualistic mannerisms, such as rocking and spinning (themselves or objects).

(9) A background of serious retardation in which islets of normal, near normal or exceptional intellectual function or skill may appear.

Not all of these criteria were acceptable without modification or addition to all members of the working party. Indeed, in the years which have elapsed since their publication, doubts about the validity of some of them have been expressed both by members of the working party and by others. To the present writer it seemed, in considering (1), for example, that the child's aloofness was not confined to his failure to form or maintain normal personal relationships. These children also show an aloofness from, and a lack of interest or participation in, reality as a whole. They take little part in our world; they live—as most of their mothers will say—' in a world of their own '. The name usually given to this phenomenon is ' withdrawal ', although in many cases the child has not so much withdrawn as failed ever to become normally involved with reality.

In the same way it is difficult to accept without qualification the description (2), which arose from acceptance of the view of Norman (1954), supported more recently by Goldfarb (1964), because it seems that to ascribe such symptoms as self-examination, or self-mutilation, or misuse of personal pronouns to a lack of awareness of the limitations of his own body is a subjective interpretation of the child's behaviour rather than a description of it. Goldfarb attributes many of the features of what he calls schizophrenic children to ' extreme defects in self-awareness '. He refers to experimental findings which, he claims, confirm that in these patients there are ' major gaps in ability to perceive, discriminate, localize and give meaning to body percepts '. There is undoubtedly some evidence of the existence of such perceptual disabilities, but to infer that they are due to a lack of integrated and stable body awareness is an assumption which seems difficult indeed to justify.

Goldfarb is convinced by what he calls ' a flood of naturalistic evidence ' that because the schizophrenic child portrays the body as ' broken, disintegrating, and lacking in intact boundaries ', therefore he is not normally aware of his own body. But is this necessarily so? Must the child's perceptual disabilities necessarily imply a lack of normal awareness of his own body? Presumably these perceptual disabilities must arise from peripheral or central sensory dysfunction. In other words, his inability to perceive a sight adequately must be due either to inability to see properly, or to inability to make a meaningful synthesis of sensory impulses arriving in the brain, or to disinclination to look properly. His peculiar representations of the body might be due to an inability accurately to perceive his own or other persons' bodies; but they might alternatively be due to a lack of interest in accurately portraying either bodies or any other aspect of reality. A withdrawn child cares little about reality, so his portrayals of the body will be but little influenced by checking against reality or by people's reactions to what he draws. It could be that the

9

child is simply not bothered by any need to make a photographic representation. Or perhaps he could be simply playing with distortions of the body in the way of modern artists. After all, Picasso and Henry Moore have produced some peculiarly distorted bodies, but nobody suggests that either of them has disturbance of body image, or even that their perception of the human body is abnormal.

Certainly there seems to be little evidence that the repeated self-directed aggression implies a lack of awareness of the child's own personal identity. On the contrary, one of the features of the syndrome appears to be a preoccupation of the child with his own body, and a tendency to seek satisfaction almost exclusively through the sensations and movements of his body. Indeed, it might be argued that many psychotic children go to very great lengths to keep their own personalities inviolate by excluding sensory stimuli or emotional overtures from the world around them. The working party's paragraph of explanation of Point (2) goes even further with this theory of lack of awareness of personal identity, suggesting that it may be responsible for the difficulties in forming personal relationships. This assumption appears to ignore many other possible explanations; for example, the child might not have been in contact with people who could form adequate relationships with him; or he might not be able to see or hear other people; or he might be too immature or too ill to be able to form personal relationships; or he might be afraid to do so because of traumatic experiences in very early life.

It seems possible that the other symptoms attributed by the working party to unawareness of personal identity could just as plausibly be ascribed to preoccupation with self to the exclusion of interest in the environment. Continual self-examination, for example, could result from such a preoccupation. Perhaps the same applies to the confusion of personal pronouns shown by some of these children. To attribute this symptom to unawareness of personal identity seems a reasonable theory at first hearing, but the following is an alternative explanation, which seems at least equally plausible. Autistic children, when they begin to speak, do so largely by way of echolalia—exact repetition of words or phrases used by others. When the child, speaking of himself, says ' he wants some more dinner ' or ' you don't want to go to bed ' he is showing echolalia, that is, he is repeating what he has heard his mother say. Now if he is withdrawn, he is not much bothered about us or about our world or our conventions. So he would care little about grammar or an accurate choice of words. Not wanting to go to bed, he would use a phrase conveying his wishes without caring too much about its form. If one is with an autistic child for long continuous periods, one can usually remember the adult's remark when the child repeats it more or less appropriately or exactly at a later time. It might be suggested that he is not so much confused about personal pronouns, as not bothered about them.

Points (4), (5) and (6) have also been criticized (Ingram, 1965) because subjective interpretations are involved. Although the objective observations described would be agreed with by the vast majority of those who have to treat these children, the interpretations expressed or implied can only be described as gratuitous. For example, does unpredictable response to sensory stimuli necessarily imply abnormal perceptual experience? How can the examiner judge that anxiety is, by the child's own premises, excessive or illogical?

Criticism might also be levelled at the use of Point (9), as it stands, as a criterion of diagnosis of the schizophrenic syndrome; for, though serious retardation usually is present in this syndrome, it is also present in many other conditions, and unless islands of intelligence are present, intellectual retardation can hardly be regarded as a legitimate criterion of the schizophrenic syndrome.

It seemed that the most important point emerging from discussions by the working party before and after publication of the ' Nine Points ', or criteria, was that one criterion was present in nearly every case, namely the first. Indeed, when psychiatrists from all over the world were asked to test the validity of the nine points in children they regarded as 'schizophrenic' or 'autistic' or 'psychotic' there were very few patients reported as not showing disturbances of emotional relationships, and this criterion emerges as probably a *sine qua non* of the syndrome.

Nearly always, the disturbance of emotional relationships takes the form of what is called 'withdrawal' or failure to be involved emotionally with people to the normal extent. Having criticized the 'Nine Points' on account of their subjective interpretations, one has to admit that usually the decision that a child is withdrawn is made on a subjective basis, that is to say, the psychiatrist says that the child is withdrawn if he himself can make no adequate rapport with him, if he gets no feeling of emotional response from the child. To the present writer, and to most psychiatrists experienced in this field, this subjective assessment has been justified through clinical experience and borne out by the subsequent behaviour and development of large numbers of cases. However, subjective assessments are difficult to quantify or classify and one has to seek for an objective criterion of withdrawal, particularly since there are a few people, among them the parents of some autistic children, who would not agree that these children are withdrawn. In fact, however, one can assess the amount of withdrawal objectively, because the extent to which a child associates with his contemporaries during free play, or joins in their games, can be measured quite simply, and in fact, the extent to which the child avoids association with other children usually tallies pretty accurately with the psychiatrist's assessment of the child's degree of withdrawal during the first interview.

If withdrawal or non-involvement is in fact the most important symptom, then the symptomatology as a whole might perhaps be considered from a different point of view. It might be suggested that the withdrawal from people is primary, the supposition being that the normal child's inclination to interest himself in reality in general depends on his relationships and identifications with people, whereas an autistic child is self-absorbed and does not make normal relationships and identifications, and, as the result, does not interest himself or seek to involve himself in the aspirations and activities of other people. At all events it seems that autistic children are nearly always withdrawn from several or many aspects of reality.

Perhaps in due course it might be advisable to revise the 'nine points', listing the essential features of the schizophrenic syndrome in childhood as follows:

(1) Withdrawal from, or failure to become involved with, reality; in particular, failure to form normal relationships with people.

(2) Serious intellectual retardation with islets of higher, or nearly normal or exceptional intellectual function or skills.

(3) Failure to acquire speech, or to maintain or improve on speech already learned, or to use what speech has been acquired for communication.

(4) Abnormal response to one or more types of sensory stimulus (usually sound).

(5) Gross and sustained exhibition of mannerisms or peculiarities of movement, including immobility and hyperkinesis, and excluding tics.

(6) Pathological resistance to change. This may be shown by:

(a) Insisting on observance of rituals in the patient's own behaviour or in those around him.

(b) Pathological attachment to the same surroundings, equipment, toys and people (even though the relationship with the person involved may be purely mechanical and emotionally empty).

(c) Excessive preoccupation with particular objects or certain characteristics of them without regard to their accepted functions.

(*d*) Severe anger or terror or excitement, or increased withdrawal, when the sameness of the environment is threatened (e.g. by strangers).

14

CHAPTER 2

CHILDHOOD SCHIZOPHRENIA

There has been considerable controversy over the use of the term 'childhood schizophrenia' or 'schizophrenic syndrome' for the group of children embraced by the above criteria, some observers being far from convinced that the disease process in these children is basically the same as that in adult schizophrenics. It is of course understandable that the parents and others who love these children would dislike to apply to them a term which carries such a gloomy prognosis (although, in fact, recent advances in the treatment of adults diagnosed as schizophrenic have given them a prognosis which is rather better, in terms of capacity for living a self-supporting life, than is the case in children diagnosed as autistic). Certainly the psychiatrist would wish to be very sure of himself before making the diagnosis and would take great pains to explain to the parents exactly what he meant. This is particularly important since there is so much confusion about what is meant by the term schizophrenia; to some people it connotes incurable mental illness, whilst others, literary persons rather than doctors, seem to use the term to imply ambivalence or mere conflict in the individual's mind. One writer recently has gone so far as to suggest that the term 'schizophrenia' should no longer be used scientifically without specific definition of what it means in the particular context (Bannister, 1968).

Medical critics who dislike the term 'childhood schizophrenia' point out that hallucinations, and even expressed delusions, are relatively uncommon in these children, especially the younger patients; they refer to the intellectual retardation which usually exists, in contrast to adult schizophrenia in which, nowadays, true dementia is not usually regarded as being common; and they emphasize that the tranquillizers are very seldom effective in treatment—again in contrast to adult schizophrenia. All these points are borne out by the present writer's experience, although such authorities as Bender maintain that drugs are effective in treatment in certain cases; indeed, Bender claims considerable success with such drugs as chlorpromazine, Frenquel (azacylonal hydrochloride), Bena-dryl, Phenergan and even LSD (lysergic acid diethylamide) (Bender and Nichtern, 1956; Bender, Faretra and Cobrinik, 1963). Similar results have been claimed by others (Bender, 1956; Faretra and Bender, 1964) though clinical experience of these drugs in Britain does not appear to have been so favour-able. Moreover, Bender maintains that electric shock treat-ment is still the treatment of choice in, and should not be withheld from, autistic children suffering from acute and severe psychotic episodes. All this, of course, corresponds with the general experience in adult schizophrenia.

Nobody has yet suggested any series of diagnostic criteria for adult schizophrenia corresponding with the ' Nine Points ' for the schizophrenic syndrome in childhood; but if any such list were to be compiled surely the most frequent and outstanding feature would be the same—namely, a difficulty in forming and maintaining personal relationships, a tendency to solitariness and withdrawal from people and the world around them. Abnormalities of speech would figure high in the list, particularly a failure to use speech for purposes of normal communication. Abnormal response to sensory stimuli would also be regarded as a common feature (witness the tendency of many adult schizophrenics to ignore or to put a false interpretation upon remarks made by other people, and the burns which used to be so frequently seen upon the legs of adult schizophrenics who tend, unless watched carefully, to stand too close to the radiator). Mannerisms and pecu-liarities of movement are the common currency of the adult schizophrenic and apparently excessive anger or terror or excitement are as frequently seen in the adult schizophrenic as in the autistic child. Nor is a slavish adherence to routine an uncommon feature of adult schizophrenia.

Rutter (1965) has expressed the view that as applied to autistic children, ' the term schizophrenia is a complete misnomer '. He suggests that ' schizophrenia can begin in childhood, but only very rarely does it begin before puberty '. This view is, of course, in flat contradiction to that of the vast majority of psychiatrists who have experience of adolescent and young adult schizophrenics (Arieti, 1959). To the present writer's knowledge, nobody has previously denied that in a very large number of adult schizophrenics there is a clear history of a morbid pre-psychotic personality, or of signs of incipient schizophrenia in adolescence or childhood. Rutter states further that ' unlike adult schizophrenia, child psychosis is frequently associated with mental subnormality . . .' It is, of course, difficult to give a scientific definition of what is meant by mental subnormality; but if failure to attain a normal score on intelligence testing is an important sign of mental subnormality then there must be a very large number indeed of adult schizophrenics who would be found, on testing, to be functioning as mentally subnormal, especially if one includes those adult schizophrenics who would refuse to co-operate adequately in testing and who might for that reason be given a very low score. Moreover, it is certain that a considerable proportion of chronic patients in hospitals for the mentally subnormal show psychotic features, most of which would usually be regarded as ' schizophrenic '.

Rutter also suggests that in childhood autism ' only rarely is there a family history of schizophrenia '. This is in marked contrast to the experience at Smiths Hospital where there are two autistic brothers in residence, and where there is another severely autistic child who has a similarly autistic brother living outside. At the same time (1st March, 1966) there was in Smiths Hospital an autistic child and her actively schizophrenic hallucinated mother. In the same hospital there were, between 1963 and 1967, no less than four autistic children with actively psychotic mothers.

Without access to the patient's history, and judging purely from the present clinical condition, it is exceedingly difficult to distinguish the autistic child who has grown up and deteriorated from the schizophrenic whose illness began in early adult life who has also deteriorated. Indeed neither the present writer nor any colleague he has consulted who has long term experience of schizophrenia can confidently make such distinction. This is confirmed by the recent work of Rabinovitch and his colleagues (1965).

Case No. 3. Jill. Admitted to Smiths Hospital aged six years six months.

Summary—Childhood schizophrenia; mother's family unstable; mother schizoid; normal early development; backwardness and withdrawal from one year; diagnosed 'deaf' and 'receptive aphasia' when four and five, but hears normally; delayed and peculiar speech, first words at four years, echolalia of odd words and phrases at six years, peculiar intonation; talent for drawing but generally backward; some improvement but presents many features of adolescent schizophrenia.

Mother's description—Ignores people and speech; temper tantrums, over-active; uses people as tools; backward, does not talk.

Family—Father, aged 45 at Jill's birth, had four children by a previous marriage. All his family are normal. He tries to treat Jill as a normal child, is very dutiful but contact is not very warm. Mother, aged 23 at the child's birth, previously married and divorced, had four sisters who were admitted to mental hospitals for varying periods. She is a withdrawn schizoid woman often near to psychotic illness who was especially withdrawn around Jill's birth and has never had a warm relationship with her. It is difficult to make emotional contact with her or secure proper co-operation. There is one brother, 21 months younger, described as difficult, asocial and withdrawn.

History—Pregnancy and labour normal, no neonatal illness. Breast fed for four months, then the milk dried up. She accepted the bottle and solid foods soon afterwards. By eight months she was feeding herself, and sitting up unaided; standing by eleven months, walking well by two years. At ten months she had a combined injection against pertussis and diphtheria. Her father thinks she went back from that time, when the parents also had business and domestic worries. She became much more disturbed after the birth of her brother when she was 21 months old. She was toilet trained by four years, but wet the bed for a few months at the age of $7\frac{1}{2}$. She failed to respond to speech and was found to have no ordinary deafness but was thought to have receptive aphasia, and to be a case of ' true congenital auditory imperception '. In addition, she was found to have temperamental peculiarities and her response to testing showed very great scatter. She went to a school for the deaf, aged four, a school for disturbed children, aged six, then for short periods to two primary schools and an E.S.N. school.

Mental state on admission—She was over-active, distractible, explored and smelt everything. She understood but ignored speech, showed echolalia but no real spontaneous speech. She ignored the children but made a very superficial contact with some adults, using them as tools. She was preoccupied with surfaces and textures, she was aggressive and had tantrums. At the age of seven she began to speak spontaneously and appropriately and she showed a tendency to try to fix the attention of adults by repetitious questioning without permitting any close relationship. Slowly, she formed a deeper relationship with the matron and with the writer, but she remained considerably withdrawn. She has a talent for drawing and has learned to read and write. At the age of $12\frac{1}{2}$ she began to attend the local secondary modern school two days a week for English and Art, continuing to attend the hospital school for other subjects. She was about four or five years retarded educationally. She could not think in abstracts or use language effectively to communicate her thoughts and wishes. She spoke in a peculiar, nasal, sing-song voice. She went through a phase of using the third person or her Christian name instead of the first personal pronoun. Her approach to the Rorschach Test at $14\frac{1}{2}$ years was rigidly obsessional and she confined her responses to the interpretation of minute details. Response to each blot consisted of a methodical enumeration of all the parts of it though a total response was hardly ever given. She showed these obsessional features in her daily life, clinging to her routines, and also had sudden crises of panic when she constantly sought reassurance about something which was said either recently or in the past. She has been preoccupied with her bodily functions, especially bowel movements, and about being too fat or too thin. Her intelligence test results are summarized in Table 1.

Physical health has been good. Neurological investigations and examinations have been consistently negative and her EEG has been consistently within normal limits.

At the age of 18 she speaks in a nasal, monotonous voice. She sits inertly and walks with a stiff, odd gait. She volunteers nothing in conversation, and her answers are short, consisting very often of, ' I don't know '. She has no ambitions or plans for her future, and she does nothing unless directed. She will work industriously all day on assigned tasks, doing beautiful sewing or handwork. She attends the patients' clubs because she is taken there, but she does not associate or converse with other patients. Asked if she has a boy friend she mentions one of the patients but she knows nothing of him except his name and does not approach or speak to him. She has had two or three phases of excitement with minor violence, but without apparent direction, in which she appeared to be aurally hallucinated and said she heard voices. She still shows obsessional rituals and her behaviour remains stereotyped.

TABLE 1

Terman Merrill			Wechsler Intelligence Scale for Children		
			Intelligence quotients		
Chronological age	Mental age	Intelligence quotient	Verbal	Performance	Full scale
6 : 8	2 : 4	37			
7 : 4	3 : 2	40		67	
7 : 10	3 : 3	39		75	
8 : 2	3 : 5	42		79	
9 : 5	4 : 10	56			
10 : 6	5 : 3	58		76	
11 : 1	5 : 5	58			
11 : 11	6 : 2	62		100	
13 : 3	6 : 10	61	63	100	74
14 : 6	7 : 6	57	69	101	83

Jill's present symptoms have altered slightly and slowly through the years, but they are in essence very similar to her childhood symptoms, and to those of typical schizophrenics in whom the illness has been first recognized in adult life; and the older she gets, and the more she deteriorates, the harder would it be to distinguish her clinical state from that of dozens of other adult schizophrenics in psychiatric hospitals.

The following case in which the illness was first diagnosed in adult life may be given as an example.

Case No. 4. Mrs C.W.

She was first seen at the age of 38 when she brought her daughter to the clinic. They were accompanied by her husband who did all the talking, Mrs W. saying not a word. The daughter was taken on for treatment at the clinic and attended irregularly for several months. Sometimes the child was brought by her father, sometimes by Mrs W. who, however, rarely spoke even when questioned directly and repeatedly. She could manage her housework quite well it seemed, and she and the child were beautifully dressed. But she co-operated very little in the child's treatment and the case-work was done with the father, who said that Mrs W. rarely had contacts with people outside the home. After a year the child was admitted to hospital. Thereafter, when the social worker visited the home she only saw the father; Mrs W. behaved oddly, thumping about upstairs and throwing her shoes against the front door.

About four years later the father died, and Mrs W. was left alone. Her visits to the daughter in hospital were very rare indeed though she often asked for her to be discharged. Eventually, she locked her door and refused admission to the psychiatric social worker and to everyone else, including the doctor. Soon afterwards she began throwing stones at the neighbours' windows and accused them of persecuting her and talking about her. The mental health officer had to break into the house and she was compulsorily admitted to hospital. There she was described as ' unwilling to talk, solitary, suspicious. Wanders off if not watched; smiles at times to herself.' She was said to show inappropriate mood, to be cold, rather emotionless, flat. She seemed unconcerned at the removal of her child. She would suddenly laugh at trivial, humourless happenings or remarks. She was deluded, believing the neighbours were persecuting her and that they had been pricking her skin with electric sparks from their upstairs windows. She was further described as being vague, her affect shallow and inappropriate. She was very preoccupied with her thoughts to the exclusion of everything else. She was diagnosed as suffering from chronic schizophrenia. Her intelligence was in the normal range.

She improved in hospital but soon relapsed after being sent home, and had to be re-admitted. This pattern has been repeated several times. She makes no attempt to contact her daughter.

This lady is the mother of Christine (Case No. 7, p. 32). She is typically schizophrenic; her daughter is not a typically autistic or schizophrenic child, but she shows many points of similarity to children who are typically autistic.

It does seem, in fact, that there are many points of clinical similarity between these ' autistic ' children and schizophrenic adults. They have the same loss of contact with reality, the same self-absorption, the same lack of sympathy and warmth, the same failure to make friends; they show the same inappropriateness of utterance and action, the same kind of failure at times to use abilities which they use easily at other times; and similar unexplained fluctuations of mood. Admittedly there are also many differences, just as there are many ways in which the thinking and behaviour of a normal child differ from that of a normal adult. For example, it is to be expected that the pathological mannerisms displayed by the child will differ from those of the adult, just as the play of a normal child differs from the activities of his elders.

These considerations, reviewed in the light of a large number of clinical cases, indicate that the clinical picture of schizophrenia, or autism, in childhood might be regarded as truly analogous to that in adults if one allowed for the effect of the schizophrenic process on the developing personality and intellect of the child. It would be expected that the earlier the disease process begins the less chance will the personality have had to become defined and stable, and the greater will be the devastation of personality and intellect produced by the disease process—this difference being seen in its most extreme form if we contrast the personality of the rigid elderly para-noiac with the formless and undeveloped personality of the young schizophrenic child. But the younger the schizophrenic adult or adolescent is, the more will he resemble one of this group of autistic children. Indeed, one could say there is no dividing line between the two, no age and no point in the development of symptomatology at which one can say, ' this is a childhood rather than an adult type of schizophrenia '.

The clinical picture, in adult schizophrenia, tends to vary with the age of onset, paranoid reactions, for example, being commoner in the older patients, ' simple ' schizophrenia commoner in the young. But a schizophrenic aged 16 shows no essential differences from one aged 15, nor is a schizophrenic (or autistic) child of seven essentially different from one aged six or five, or even two. Nevertheless, one accepts a wide variation in the clinical picture just as one includes the catatonic and the florid hebephrenic within the schizophrenic group in the adult (Bleuler, 1952). Indeed, one of the most striking features of adult, as well as juvenile schizophrenics, is that no two cases are exactly alike. One might almost suggest that every case of schizophrenia consti-tutes a syndrome *sui generis*, and that, although we can roughly divide all schizophrenics into certain groups, in every case the pathology must be different, because no two human minds— not even those of identical twins—can be exactly alike. Possibly the mistake we make is in thinking of childhood autism and adult schizophrenia as diseases. If we contented ourselves by saying that autistic children and adult schizo-phrenics have in common certain abnormal ways of reacting, this controversy might become less acute and less traumatic.

CHAPTER 3

DEFENCE MECHANISMS AGAINST
INTOLERABLE REALITY

Goldfarb (1964) has emphasized the contention that '. . . each schizophrenic child's adaptive abberations are seen as highly individualized accommodations to the very special requirements of his psycho-social environment '. His views appear to coincide with the present writer's suggestion that the schizophrenic withdrawal in every case is to be regarded as one of a series of alternative, or consecutive, or coexistent mechanisms through which the child seeks to adjust himself to his environment.

From time to time, the reality situation with which any child is confronted is, for him, in his present state, unacceptable or even intolerable. Faced with the unwanted reality situation, the individual may attempt to deal with it by one of four methods: firstly, he may seek to alter or influence the situation by appropriate action—he flees, or he fights, or he strives appropriately to cope. Secondly, he may try to prevent this and similar unwanted situations by making reality less unpredictable. If one knows what time the train will leave, or when the man is coming in for supper, or under what circumstances one's opponent will deliver his left hook, then life becomes easier, more tolerable, less frightening. So the wife tries to make the man come in at a regular time each evening; the commuter supports attempts to get trains to run to schedule; the boxer tries to keep the initiative in the fight so as to impose his own pattern and thus prevent the opponent unleashing the left hook, except when he is prepared to counter it. This method of controlling reality is practised universally by normal children as by adults. But the disturbed child uses it to a pathological extent, so that it then constitutes an abnormal means of coping with reality. For the child seeks to control all or most aspects of reality-as-it-affects-him by *imposing rituals* and by trying to prevent variation in any aspect of his environment, be it people, or toys, or living space or furniture. If he can 'monotonize' the environment so that nothing changes, reality becomes less frightening or demanding, and on these terms he can cope with it, more or less. When this attempt fails, as it usually will, he may be driven to the third alternative defence: he may attempt to make reality acceptable by *distortion*, that is to say, by self-deception, fantasy, delusion or hallucination. In this way he can change reality-as-he-sees-it, so that it becomes tolerable, so that it shows him in a better light or removes his frustrations or fulfils his aspirations, or explains his failures. This, again, is probably a normal defence mechanism provided it is not carried to excess. Only by practising a certain amount of self-deception could the majority of the British people have sustained their determination to fight in 1940. The Christian and the dialectical materialist both need and are sustained by their respective faiths, but they cannot both be right. One or the other must be labouring under a certain amount of useful self-deception. Only if used to an excessive degree can the process be called abnormal.

Finally, if none of these mechanisms succeeds in protecting him from intolerable reality, his only course is to adopt the fourth mechanism of defence—that is, to withdraw; to try to exclude reality (or at least those aspects of reality which he cannot control, normally or by 'monotonization' or distortion), and live as far as possible within himself, ignoring or failing to respond to sensory stimuli or to make emotional relationships. In later chapters an attempt will be made to show that withdrawal is also a normal defence mechanism, used by every human being to a great extent, and only to be regarded as abnormal when it prejudices the biological survival of the individual as it does

25

in the autistic child and the schizophrenic adult. (In the adult there is, of course, a fifth method of escape, namely, suicide. But this alternative does not occur to the autistic child; no-one has ever told him that he can escape from it all by cutting his throat, and indeed the idea of his own death does not occur to him—as is evident from the way in which he will run out into the road or climb along high ledges without apparent fear.)

Very often, of course, and especially in children diagnosed as ' autistic ' or ' schizophrenic ', elements of all three abnormal processes are present: withdrawal, plus distortion, plus ritualistic attempts at control of reality (as well as, perhaps, tentative and abortive efforts at normal attempts to cope); and this partly accounts for the variation in symptomatology. We may see a child in a moderately severe stage of his illness who is still attempting to control reality by rituals and by insisting on sameness, and who shows tantrums when these attempts are thwarted, whilst at the same time he is distorting reality in his fantasies—which may be expressed as delusions—and, at times, withdrawing more or less completely from reality, which, therefore, no longer controls his thoughts and actions.

Case No. 5. John. Admitted to Smiths Hospital aged six years three months

Summary—Parents depressed around the time of birth, ambivalent and tense towards the child; withdrawal, ritualism and obsessional mannerisms; improving under treatment.

Mother's description—Inadequate speech; slow developer; odd mannerisms; clings to rituals, panics if they are upset.

History—Pregnancy; mother was depressed, with constant vomiting. Normal delivery, birth weight $7\frac{1}{2}$ lb. Mother aged 27, father aged 32. Breast fed for six months, an easy feeder. Weaned to cup and spoon at six months with no difficulty. At 18 months began refusing solids and new foods, insisted on a strict ritual at meals. This persisted until a few weeks after admission. Sat up at one year, crawled at 18 months, walked at two years. Mother tried early to train him to the pot but he would not co-operate until almost a year old. At three years he could only say ' mama ' and ' dada '. At $3\frac{1}{2}$ years he became preoccupied with flicking the pages of books past his nose. At three years nine months a paediatrician described him as ' ? mentally retarded, peculiar, egocentric, but not withdrawn ', and at four years one month as ' odder still, obsessional about routines in his life. Used my hand to place blocks on form board. Speech full of expression but only jargon. Uses proper phrases when worked up without relation to the situation. Shouts them frantically ', and at three years ten months as, ' I now think John is psychotic, though peculiar, due to his obsessionalism and not being markedly withdrawn '. He was described by the writer, at four years five months as ' withdrawn with prominent mannerisms and obsessionalism. Home treatment would be possible if not for mother's disturbance over husband ', and at four years ten months as ' showing strong obsessional features. Carries an old bit of jersey round as a fetish. Poor articulation, frequent repetition of phrases, fear of anything new, and odd mannerisms. Ambivalent to mother, sadistic and demanding cuddling. Mother could not conceal resentment '. At that time his mother said that he was talking better but still not making proper sentences or asking questions. Whereas previously he had been most unwilling to go out among people he would now do so, though he soon wanted to come home. He would not play with new toys unless mother was present. The mother was now receiving encouragement and explanations from the general practitioner and from the writer, who described him at five years nine months as ' less obsessional, less over-active, more friendly, less withdrawn, more capable of normal play, less than normally able to associate with other children, but will join in if they take the lead ', and at $6\frac{1}{2}$ years as ' playing by himself and with the same toy for days. Does not use knife or fork, refuses to chew his food. Dry by day, wet by night. Insists on pot instead of WC '. On admission to Smiths Hospital at the age of six years nine months he was a passive child who went without protest with adults, showed echolalia with frequent appropriate remarks, named objects, showed no attempt to play with children or material presented to him, was clean and tidy and resented any disturbance in his routine. He had learned the alphabet and was beginning to show interest in reading. At the end of March, 1962 he showed very little echolalia, co-operated much more, being willing to sit down and do painting or play games with adults. Questions were answered briefly but correctly. His mother was now coming into the hospital on one afternoon a week, spending most of that time with John. He was still withdrawn and peculiar but considerably improved. His mental age on testing rose from three years three months on 20.9.61 to four years two months on 13.11.61. ' In six months he has achieved a twelve months' improvement in functioning.' His EEG on 10.11.61 showed stable alpha rhythm and no definite abnormality except paroxysms of non-classical spike and wave complexes in all leads bilaterally on over breathing. Subsequent EEG's showed no change except that it was no longer possible to elicit the spike and wave complexes described above. A great deal of work was done by the psychiatric social worker with the parents, who became progressively more confident, keener to have John at home and more critical of the hospital.

By the winter of 1965 he had left hospital and was attending a day school for the educationally subnormal. His voice was still peculiar, his manner a little odd, but he asked and answered questions appropriately and was keen to join in other children's games. He was still very sensitive to any hostility or harshness, becoming more inert and withdrawn, but he was making some progress at school, he had two good friends (girls) and showed much more spontaneity and normal interest in his surroundings.

Abnormal Attempts to Control Reality

This process is most easily observed when schizophrenic deviation begins in childhood, as opposed to infancy or adult life. Usually there is, in the early stages, an attempt to alter or control reality by normal methods which, as they fail, become increasingly abnormal. Thus, normal aggressiveness and appropriate anger are replaced by impulsive violence and tantrums; normal fear gives way to unreasoning panics. Ordinary tidiness becomes excessive; normal routines become obsessive rituals. The child seems to attempt to monotonize the environment, to pick out certain aspects of reality which are tolerable, and which he can control, and to try to fill his life with these to the exclusion of all else (*see* Case Nos. 1, 2 and 6). Thus he may play exclusively with one particular toy or at one repetitive game, or insist on exactly the same form of greeting on each occasion, exactly the same wording of a phrase used frequently by his mother, the same food, the same ritual at the table or at the toilet. A slight deviation from the ritual may provoke the wildest possible tantrums, with violence or self-injury. The most unpredictable elements of reality are people, and one of the functions of these rituals seems to be to control the person involved and to prevent him from altering the environment. If the child finds a remark or a situation, particularly one involving his mother, which is reassuring and which he feels strengthens his control of reality, he may continue to repeat that remark or to prolong that situation interminably. A related symptom is the tendency, shown by so many children in whom the schizophrenic deviation is less severe or is later in onset, repeatedly to ask questions to which the child knows the answers.

Case No. 6. Peter. Admitted to Smiths Hospital aged five years five months

Summary—Psychotic family history, parents' relationships complicated by the war; neonatal illness; retardation, failure to form relationships or to speak; restlessness, wandering, mannerisms, rituals, tantrums; EEG shows atypical spike and waves; improvement under treatment.

History—Mother was in bed with nephritis and high blood pressure for several weeks during the pregnancy. She had pethidine and then chloroform at labour which was forceps-assisted. Birth weight 9½ lb. He was slightly jaundiced soon after birth and according to the mother, a few days later his skin peeled. He was oedematous, sweated excessively and cried continuously. In hospital the diagnosis was ' dehydration fever '. After 14 days in hospital he improved, but for the first five or six weeks he cried excessively, especially at night, to mother's extreme distress. He then slowly became placid, sleeping a great deal. He was fed by expressed milk for two weeks and then at the breast for four weeks, then transferred to the bottle because mother could not tolerate breast feeding. He was weaned without trouble at five months. He smiled early, sat at one year, stood at two years, walked at two and a quarter. He never crawled but sat inertly wherever he was put. At the age of about four he began to be restless and to wander away, often for considerable distances. He ignored other children, and the mother felt he did not make an adequate response to her although he screamed whenever she spoke to anyone else. He was preoccupied with water-closets and with shiny surfaces.

On admission to hospital he could say only a few words, his gait was poorly co-ordinated, he ignored the other children. He had a mannerism of rubbing his upper lip against the number-plates of cars. He would not settle down to sleep at night but was sleepy during the day. He had a great deal of individual treatment and began to form relationships with the doctor and the matron, and then with other members of staff. He began to speak, but in a peculiar nasal voice with poor articulation and a tendency to stutter, both of which have slowly improved. He was very jealous of other children but he slowly began to play with them and to form relationships. His social maturity improved rapidly but it was difficult to get him to co-operate in group activities. He attempted to fix the attention of adults by repetitive questioning, and he insisted on the same set routine for every procedure or game or greeting. If thwarted he had tantrums. He became preoccupied with the gramophone and then with the records. Though at first he made little attempt to read in school he learned to recognize the names of tunes from the record labels, and from this derived an interest in reading. He was reading well by the age of seven and a half. He developed a great thirst for knowledge, and began to co-operate well in school. At the age of ten he began to attend the local junior school and though he had to be excluded for a time for bad behaviour he resumed after a few weeks. In the hospital his behaviour became more controlled, his mannerisms decreased, his speech improved and his insistence on rituals diminished. Unfortunately he tended to regress when he was in his mother's company, and at this stage she was obviously severely disturbed by the child's illness. Intensive psychiatric treatment of the mother began when Peter was ten. At 11, Peter went to a boarding school for E.S.N. children where he at first did well. His behaviour deteriorated very much during the holidays but, although it was difficult to persuade him to work on occasions, his behaviour at school was good. He still could not tolerate mother's interest in a third party and sought to monopolize her attention by repetitive questions. He associated more with children at school but did not make friends either there or at home. At the age of 14 he was about three years retarded at school. The results of intelligence tests are shown in Table 2. At the age of seven years he had a

TABLE 2

Terman Merrill		Weschler Intelligence Scale for Children	
Chronological age	Intelligence quotient	Chronological age	Intelligence quotient
4	68	7	67
6	75	8	65
7	62	10	76
8	73	14	76
9	69		
14	68		

series of what appeared to be petit mal attacks and at that time, and again when aged eight, his EEG showed atypical spike and wave activity. He had no reported fits of any kind for five years and at age 14 his EEG showed no abnormality, but a further EEG two years later showed one short high voltage bilateral non-focal paroxysm of non-classical spike and wave, and about this time he had a major fit—his first for seven years. Since then he has grand mal fits about twice a year.

At this time, however, his behaviour began to deteriorate in school. He wandered away, got up in the middle of the night and did little work. He was given large doses of Melleril in order to sedate him, but this made him sleep excessively. Eventually he had to be admitted to hospital (aged 16). He attended the local day school for a time but soon began to abscond and steal. He had to be kept in a locked ward where he would do no work unless forced. He made no real friendships, was self-absorbed, auto-erotic, muttered to himself and was inert and listless. However, he responded to an active programme of occupation, individual schooling, social activity, personal supervision and encouragement by the staff and frequent visits by his mother. He became more socially aware, absconded less frequently, showed fewer mannerisms and associated more freely. At the height of his disturbance, aged

17, his W.I.S.C. I.Q. had deteriorated to 53 and the psychologist was ' left with the impression of some frank thought disorder '. At the age of 20 he is still very immature and unable to make relationships except those which a five or six year old makes with familiar adults. He has few interests except ' pop ' records, no mature plans for his own future, no inclination to work. Ordinary social pressures mean very little to him but he likes to attend the Roman Catholic Church, where the ritual of the services appeals to him. He has some interest in the opposite sex, as shown by sexually coloured remarks about ' pop ' singers and girls with long hair, and by hugging older woman quite violently; but he makes no normal approaches to girls, and he is so infantile and so unable to share or appreciate other people's feelings or interests that neither girls nor boys will have much to do with him.

Case No. 7. Christine. Admitted to Smiths Hospital on 22.11.56 aged ten years three months

Summary—Severely disturbed personality, schizoid and hysterical features; precocious early development; insidious onset with tantrums beginning at five; facile, superficial and sensuous contact with adults but no deep emotional relationship; five epileptic fits, abnormal EEG; average intelligence, educational retardation; improvement under treatment in spite of loss of parents.

Mother's complaints—Tantrums, misbehaviour at school; cuddles up to strange adults in the park.

Family—Mother was aged 30 at the child's birth. She has never answered questions or co-operated in Christine's treatment, remaining almost mute at interview and refusing to open her door to workers from the hospital or Children's Department. For at least five years she has been in and out of mental hospital and is a chronic paranoid schizophrenic who makes irregular contact with Christine (Case No. 4). Father, an engineer, was 40 at her birth and died when Christine was 14. He always tried to conceal his wife's illness, to withhold information and to pretend all was well with the child. Both parents denied family history of mental illness but their evidence is suspect.

History—Christine was first referred at the age of six because of ' disgusting habits, over-activity and tantrums at school '. She showed off and exhibited her body, hugged adults indiscriminately, but made no real contact with other children. No school would keep her. She is an only child, born after eight years of marriage. Pregnancy was normal, birth weight $8\frac{1}{2}$ lb. She was not breast fed because mother did not wish to feed. No serious illnesses, but one epileptic fit before admission. A quiet, placid baby but became mischievous and had tantrums from three years. All milestones early, she could read before starting school.

Mental state—On admission she was superficially cheerful and serene, but, though she sought physical contact, kissing and fondling from adults, they felt that she made no real emotional contact. Indeed, her physical overtures embarrassed the staff who tended to reject her on that account. This tendency has improved steadily as the staff have learned to accept her and have formed relationships with her which are as close as she will permit, but she remains insensitive to their feelings and embarrasses them by demonstrations of affection in public. She asks repetitive questions, though these have become more sensible and appropriate through the years. The object of her ceaseless prattle appears to be to fix the attention of the adult concerned, from whom she seeks to obtain sensuous gratification without permitting a real relationship. With children, at first she made no relationship at all but later she made superficial relationships—all her emotional reactions are superficial and facile. Many of her replies were irrelevant, for example; Question: ' How do you get on with mother? ' Answer: ' I love kippers ', or, Question: ' Tell me about your daddy ', Answer: ' Daddy's dead; isn't that a lovely dog? ' Her insensitivity to the world around her and her inappropriate behaviour is exemplified by her demanding three cheers for the matron of the hospital from the children at the local secondary modern school during general assembly. None of the children, of course, had ever heard of the matron, but they responded unanimously to this riotous invitation. Christine smiles and asks riddles but has no humour.

Summary of intelligence tests—Her I.Q. has varied from 93 in 1955 to 110 in 1962 on the Terman Merrill Scale, and has been consistently around 100 on the W.I.S.C. Her main handicap is still in critical thinking. She has difficulty in detecting verbal absurdities and sometimes gives completely inappropriate answers when asked to interpret a picture or complete a simple story. She cannot distinguish between the relevant and the irrelevant.

Physical health—She has maintained very good physical health. She had single epileptic fits in 1956, 1957 and 1958, but of recent years (since 1962), fits have increased in frequency. Her EEG in 1956 was 'abnormal and of a type which is often associated with an organic lesion', being grossly irregular and showing high voltage alpha activity, of higher voltage on the right than on the left, with numerous high and medium sharp waves on both sides, more often on the left than on the right, and most marked in the left temporo-parietal region. In 1957 the record showed less abnormality, but there was less evidence of one-sidedness. In 1961 the EEG record showed 'a high voltage rhythmic activity with dominant alpha rhythm of 8 to 9 c/s. Slow activity of much lower voltage occurs as a non-specific background only, and at no time displaces the alpha rhythm. No asymmetric or focal features were seen'. The record was regarded as probably within normal limits for her age group.

Progress—In 1965 she was substantially unchanged. There were no abnormal physical signs. She relied on rituals to control her life, on riddles and conundrums and stupid repetitive questions to control conversations with adults. She had temper tantrums when thwarted, showed increasingly frequent major epileptic attacks—24 in 1964—which seem to be emotionally precipitated and in which she does not hurt herself. She asks occasionally after her mother but shows no apparent depths of emotion when told her mother will not (or cannot) visit. A middle-aged man visits her regularly in hospital. He would like to take her out and marry her, and Christine would go with him if allowed to, but her relationship with him is hopelessly superficial and immature.

A feature of both these cases was the constantly repeated neutral questions through which the child precludes advances into his own private world by his companion, yet maintains a contact with him over which the child has control. Continual chatter, apparently designed to keep the therapist at bay, is of course a familiar symptom in other disturbed, but not necessarily psychotic, children whom we see in the clinics, and is in turn to be distinguished from the constant asking of questions by the normal but anxious four-year-old who needs for the time being to fix the adult's attention on himself. The excessive anxiety, temper tantrums or fear, which are common in the autistic child at this stage, are usually provoked by threatened failure of the attempt to control the environment through such expedients as these, or the imposition of rituals. Abnormal fear of strangers is a related feature, and those who do best in caring for such children are steady, placid, reliable people whose responses do not vary.

These attempts to control reality by increasingly abnormal methods constitute some of the earliest symptoms in children showing the schizophrenic syndrome, particularly in those aged 5–10 years. As they in turn fail, the clinical picture changes, because now the patient has either to distort reality or to withdraw from it.

Distortion of Reality

The process of distortion of reality is observed less frequently in the autistic child than in the adult schizophrenic. The commonest manifestations of distortion are delusions and hallucinations; these are not often observed in autistic children although they are not infrequent in schizophrenic adolescents. Moreover, the younger the age of onset of autistic symptoms the less likely is the child to give indications of the content of underlying fantasy. However, since one of the features of this kind of illness is difficulty in communication, the patient will be unable or unwilling to tell anybody about his fantasies, and one can only infer that such fantasies are occurring from the child's general behaviour. Their drawings, at any rate in the younger patients, lack imaginative content but this could be due to absence of any ability or urge to communicate what they imagine. Alternatively, this, and the distortions of human bodies in the drawings, have been attributed to perceptual disabilities, as discussed above, or to absence of desire to observe or to portray accurately. Some of the children have a facility for playing so-called imaginative games, but the more severely affected do not appear to do so nearly as much as normal children. One presumes that the sudden changes of mood or activity, independent of what is going on around them, must be associated with some thought process, and we know from adult and adolescent schizophrenics that day dreams and fantasies, so-called ' dereistic thinking ', occupy much of their time. But their fantasies, like our own, are concerned with or based on reality—or rather on reality as they comprehend it. The autistic child has a very small interest in, and therefore a small comprehension of, reality. For this reason the content of his fantasies must be very much reduced in scope. When an ordinary child is said to be ' day dreaming ' he is either weaving fantasies about his own role in the world, the real world as he comprehends it, or else he is simply thinking about his own sensations, his own activities, his own problems, his own aspirations in the real world. The autistic child, because of the very restricted world in which he lives, has very little upon which to base his fantasies or his thoughts. Moreover, because he has very little urge to participate or advance in the real world, his need for fantasies about his own role therein must be very small. The assumption that autistic children have a rich fantasy life is, therefore, not proven, and open to some doubt. When they have temper tantrums, or sudden changes of mood and activity, this could be because people and their conventions and standards of behaviour are of little or no interest to these children who therefore have no desire to control or modify their behaviour unless it makes them uncomfortable or anxious.

All in all, such evidence as there is seems to point to a diminution rather than an increase in the content of fantasy as compared with normal children (although the time spent in day dreaming is much more), and to a much diminished liability to delusions and hallucinations as compared with the schizophrenic adult or adolescent. One surmises that if the tendency to distort reality is less in autistic children than in schizophrenic adults, it may be because such a child's involvement with, and conviction of and interest in, reality is much less than that of the adult, so that his need to distort it by fantasies and delusions is less pressing. Moreover, the process of withdrawal is so much easier for him that he tends to resort to it rather than to distortion.

Withdrawal from (or Non-involvement with) Reality

Most of the mothers of our patients tell us, ' he lives in a world of his own '. By this they mean that their children are self-absorbed, preoccupied with their own bodies, their movements and sensations, and with inanimate objects which for the most part they use in a way which we regard as inappropriate. Above all, these children have no interest or very little interest in people except as ' machines ' which will provide them with what they need, as the bringers of physical comfort or exhilaration in cuddle or acrobatic games, as providers of food and similar basic needs, or as openers of doors or drivers of cars. The term ' withdrawal ' is not always appropriate because many of these children seem never to have become truly involved with reality from the beginning. Only in cases in which the child ceases to involve himself with reality is the term withdrawal accurately used. With this caveat, however, one can continue to use the term withdrawal since it has now become traditional.

The withdrawal from, or non-involvement with, people is an essential and fundamental part of the autistic process and explains the child's failure to form normal personal relationships. These children therefore find it easiest to concern themselves with neutral objects which they can control and which, unlike people, make no demands on them. One becomes used to seeing schizophrenic children whose chief interest in life is a piece of rag, or a piece of plastic tape, or the remnants of an old teddy bear, or an old jersey, and there is no end to the variety of objects which they may adopt as their inanimate companions (Case No. 8). Only occasionally, when the illness is in its early stages, or when the child has shown some improvement, do they show any real interest in animals, which, after all, are only a little less unpredictable than human beings. Machines and appliances, on the other hand, make no demands, and indeed the child can usually control them to some extent. So the patient may be preoccupied for long periods with switches, locks, water closets or spinning tops (Case Nos. 1 and 6). This interest in machines or gadgets is, of course, very reminiscent of the schizoid adult who prefers machines to people.

Case No. 8. Bill. *Admitted to Smiths Hospital aged seven years*

Summary—Childhood autism; normal development up to 18 months then withdrawal; restless, hyperactive, not communicating spontaneously; improvement whilst cared for by mother substitute.

Mother's description—Solitary, does not make relationships, especially with children; does not use language to communicate, but occasionally produces an inappropriate adult phrase; spends most of his time jumping up and down on one spot, will not settle to any activity.

History—Mother 40 at child's birth. Normal pregnancy but admitted to hospital for anaemia in the eighth month. Birth precipitate. Weight 8 lb., no injuries. No neonatal illness. Breast fed satisfactorily for nine months. He had measles and mumps and at about ten months was said to have Bornholm's disease, the acute symptoms lasting only about a week. He had gamma globulin injections at eight months in an effort to ward off measles. At 18 months he fell from his high chair and hit his head on a concrete floor. He is said to have been semi-conscious for four hours. No apparent after-effects. He walked alone at ten months and was using phrases by 18 months. Until this time the most forward child for his age in this family, he now began to be over active and took less interest in people. Appropriate spontaneous speech got less though he would still repeat phrases at times and would also say inappropriate adult phrases as well as incomprehensible noises. He ' seemed to withdraw into a world of his own ', making no approach to other children or to his parents, and began to show compulsive behaviour with rituals. At the age of six years he was described by the psychiatrist at The Maudsley Hospital, to which he was admitted, as ' jumping up and down in the same place or running around up and down the tennis court. Fits of uncontrollable crying. Only repetitive phrases under conditions of emotion; long periods of abstraction; repetitive behaviour; a phase of standing everything on end; spinning objects; recently twisting bits of cottonwool together and tearing bits of paper, and biting pieces out of his gloves; no contact with activities of other children in the family; appeared happy and cheerful '; I.Q. remained between 44 to 50.

On admission to Smiths Hospital aged seven he was very withdrawn, sucked his fingers and shook one hand to and fro for long periods. There was no spontaneous recognizable speech, but he whispered to himself. He stared straight in front of him, was preoccupied with a piece of cottonwool and fought any attempt to take it away from him. He would sit at the table and feed himself. He was always wet, and soiled occasionally. He was given a high grade defective woman as nurse-maid. She gave him intensive individual attention for three years, by the end of which he would say anything or answer questions at her prompting. He had a real relationship with her and was beginning to play with other children, including his siblings when on holiday. He would dress and undress himself and was clean and dry, but he showed visual avoidance and would not mix with the other children or co-operate in school. Since the nurse-maid's departure when he was 11 he has made no further progress, and at 12 years he was rather more withdrawn. At the age of 15 Bill presents a picture indistinguishable to the present writer from that of the young adult schizophrenic. He is inert and very difficult to occupy, mostly he is placid with a habitual smile; he can be persuaded to answer appropriately but for the most part uses echolalia as a response; he associates hardly at all with the other children even though he has known some of them for several years, and, if left to himself, he spends much of his time and energy in psychotic mannerisms, mostly truncated survivals of those he showed in childhood and resembling more and more those of the adult schizophrenic.

Psychological testing was not possible at 12 years though he could perform on the Seguin Form Board at a 5 : 9 level and could repeat six digits. All physical investigations have proved negative. He had five EEG's at The Maudsley and Smiths Hospitals, all of which were considered within normal limits.

Are Autism and Schizophrenia properly regarded as diseases?

It seems that the symptomatology of childhood autism (and perhaps of adult schizophrenia too) becomes less obscure if we have in mind this concept of the altered relationship with reality as probably the essential feature of the illness.

It might be said, if one dared to exaggerate in order to illustrate a suggestion, that one of the chief obstacles to the understanding of the nature of schizophrenia is a medical education; the reason being that doctors are trained to think in terms of diseases, each with a pathology and, hopefully, a treatment. So modern psychiatry, which was based primarily on the medical (and, in particular, the neurological) training of men like Charcot and Freud, still has to cope with the assumption that psychiatric disturbances, like physical diseases, are due to anatomical lesions caused by heredity, by poisoning or infection, by growth, by physical trauma or by physical degeneration in the tissues concerned. The fact that minor psychiatric upsets can be caused by emotional effects of environmental changes has been obvious since the beginning of time. But medical science has been most unwilling to accept that major psychiatric upsets can be so caused; indeed, some psychiatrists hardly accept it to this day.

The neurological basis of modern psychiatry also explains why, until recently, we have sought to divide patients into concise diagnostic categories like hysteria, obsessive-compulsive neurosis, reactive depression, endogenous depression, and schizophrenia (the latter being further sub-divided into the catatonic, the hebephrenic, the paraphrenic, the 'simple' and so on).

Adolph Meyer was perhaps the first to realize the unsuitability of this approach in psychiatry, and divided patients into 'reaction types'. As time went on, more and more psychiatrists realized that very few patients fitted nicely into any of the diagnostic categories. They began to talk of schizo-affective states, implying that a patient was suffering from two 'diseases', namely schizophrenia and depression, but later contenting themselves with describing patients as showing features of both schizophrenia and depressive reactions. They saw that patients suffering from organic pathologies in the central nervous system, including post-concussional syndrome, very often reacted neurotically or with depression; they began to talk of the relative importance of the reactive (or depressive) elements, as opposed to the endogenous element, in a given case of depression; and, nowadays, they even speak of 'functional overlay' or 'hysterical elements' in schizophrenia, or suggest that certain patients may be 'using their depression hysterically'.

At the present time there seems to be a tendency to reject the traditional sub-divisions of schizophrenia. Only a very small proportion of patients are diagnosed as 'catatonic,' for example, and the diagnosis 'simple' schizophrenia has also become unpopular (Bannister, 1968). Nowadays, patients are diagnosed as schizophrenic without any attempt to categorize them further—largely, it seems, because most of them show features of more than one of the recognized sub-divisions. (The tendency has, of course, been increased by the effects of modern drugs, which modify the clinical picture so that florid schizophrenic symptomatology is less often seen.) As a result of all this, an increasing number of psychiatrists hesitate to make a traditional diagnosis, preferring to give a formulation which takes into account the patients' hereditary constitution, his previous experiences, his resulting personality, and the way in which that personality is now trying to cope with his present life situation. Only by such an assessment does the modern psychiatrist consider he has enough leads to enable him to treat the patient appropriately. Words like schizophrenia and autism and depression will

41

still be used, of course, but more and more they are recognized as describing not diseases but symptoms or reaction-patterns or processes.

What seems to be happening in autistic and schizophrenic patients is that they find their real life situation for some reason so intolerable that they cannot maintain a normal relationship with reality and therefore need to distort it or withdraw from it. The altered relationship with reality is, therefore, the essential basis of the disturbance.

Thus, the age at which the schizophrenic (or autistic) process begins seems to be of crucial importance in determining symptomatology; for on this largely depends the type of altered relationship with reality which the patient will undergo (Despert, 1947). Thus, if we may grossly over-simplify, paranoia, coming on as a rule in middle life, may be seen as the attempt of an organized personality to present, to itself and to the world around it, a plausible yet creditable explanation of a life situation the truth of which the patient finds intolerable, even though he remains, except for his delusional system, in firm contact with reality. In the paraphrenic, a less well organized personality may need the support of hallucinations to bolster an explanation of reality which his peace of mind demands, and his contact with reality is weak enough for his delusions and hallucinations to be acceptable to him. In hebephrenia, beginning at a rather younger age, contact with reality is even more impaired, and thought processes are even less liable to checking by reality, so that they become chaotic. In the catatonic, contact with reality is variable, and the patient may alternate between a complete withdrawal from reality and an attempt impulsively and violently to alter it. Simple schizophrenia tends to begin at a much younger age, and its outstanding feature is withdrawal from reality. Finally, in the autistic child, withdrawal dominates the clinical picture. In fact, the earlier the schizophrenic process begins the greater is the element of withdrawal likely to be.

Moreover, the earlier the withdrawal begins the easier it is to maintain, and the smaller the impact which reality makes upon the personality. Thus the urge to conform to reality, and the desire to alter it, is minimal. The very young schizophrenic has not known reality long enough to have a stake in it—it is less essential to him; and the schizophrenic child is even less committed to reality than his adolescent or young adult fellow sufferer.

The extent of the child's withdrawal depends on the degree to which he can tolerate reality. The autistic child will tend to withdraw more completely from those aspects of reality which are most difficult to control, that is, from people. He shrinks from any sort of emotional contact, he is entirely self-centred and he has no sympathy. This withdrawal from people is of course the most important diagnostic point. Not only does it dominate the history, not only can it be seen in the home, in the school, and in the clinic, but—most important of all—it can be felt by the examiner. One has no proper rapport with these children; one feels cold and emotionally uninvolved with them. When they laugh one feels no sympathetic gaiety. When they cry one's concern is somehow impersonal.

Making the diagnosis of this symptom of withdrawal or non-involvement is not, therefore, simply an intellectual process. It depends partly on the examiner's experience and partly on his emotions. The physician has to know exactly how much emotional rapport he can expect to make with a child of this patient's age. He has to diagnose the schizophrenic process from the emotional feel of the patient as compared with the emotional feel of the normal infant. To suggest that the most important clinical diagnostic feature of the disease process is the emotional reaction which it provokes in the examiner may seem to be unscientific, yet all experienced psychiatrists draw on their emotions to a very considerable extent in diagnosing both schizophrenia and depression in the adult. If the emotional reaction of the examiner is to constitute so important a factor in diagnosis then, of course, there is an increased liability to error, and the clinician can assess his own reliability in this respect only by following many patients through their illnesses. Yet it is remarkable how seldom those with much experience of this condition differ on a particular case.

AN HYPOTHESIS TO ACCOUNT FOR CLINICAL FEATURES

The Altered Relationship with Reality

At this point it may perhaps be appropriate to put forward an hypothesis which may in part explain the resemblance between the clinical features of childhood autism and adult schizophrenia.

It is suggested that all the various types of schizophrenic patients—the paraphrenics, the hebephrenics, the catatonics, the simple schizophrenics, the autistic children, the schizoid defectives, the patients suffering from the schizophrenic syndrome or Kanner's or Mahler's or Heller's syndromes—can be included in the schizophrenic group because they have in common the fundamental, the essential psychological abnormality of the schizophrenic process, namely an altered relationship with reality.

According to this hypothesis, schizophrenic reactions are the ultimate defence against intolerable reality; they develop in people for whom reality as they perceive it is, if not intolerable, at least so unattractive as to inhibit active participation in it. Their personalities are so vulnerable that they cannot cope with the environment as they experience it. This vulnerability may declare itself at any time of life. It may be entirely constitutional (and could be so severe that even slightly adverse environmental factors would provoke a schizophrenic reaction), or it may be produced or enhanced by disease or trauma. The disease could be hereditary or acquired, the trauma could be physical or emotional. For example, a child might have no excessive constitutional predisposition to schizophrenia, yet he might develop a schizophrenic reaction because he was so severely subnormal—due to, say, phenyl-ketonuria—as to have no resources to cope adequately with reality; or because, being blind or deaf or grossly defective—due, for example, to meningitis in infancy—the reality he experiences is so frustrating or so frightening or so unrewarding as to be intolerable (Creak 1951, 1952).

It is suggested that, with the exception of the altered relationship with reality and the symptoms arising from it, all the manifestations described as criteria of the schizophrenic syndrome can occur in conditions other than schizophrenia. Rituals, bizarre mannerisms, intellectual retardation, tantrums, pathological anxiety, all these are commonly seen in various neurotic or psychotic disorders. The hypothesis implies that the children (and perhaps the adults also) whom we diagnose as schizophrenics are in fact those who have an altered relationship with reality, no matter what other symptoms they may show. It is this altered relationship which is responsible for the essential clinical features of schizophrenia; although the type of altered relationship will depend on a variety of circumstances, for example, hereditary constitution, age of onset, and degree of stress or support from the environment.

The combination, in varying proportions, of the four defence mechanisms, that is, normal and abnormal attempts at control of reality, distortion of reality and withdrawal from reality, accounts largely for the infinitely varied clinical picture in children diagnosed as suffering from schizophrenia or the schizophrenic syndrome or childhood autism.

CHAPTER 4

THE AETIOLOGY OF AUTISM

With regard to the genesis of schizophrenic or autistic symptoms in childhood, there have been two main schools of thought. One view is that such symptoms are produced, or at any rate precipitated, principally by emotional stresses, by environmental difficulties to which the child responds by withdrawal and by the other autistic symptoms described above. The other view has been that autism is due to anatomical lesions in the central nervous system with or without associated lesions elsewhere. More recently, evidence has been produced of physiological, that is, metabolic disturbance in these children, which has been suggested as the cause of their illness. There is also, of course, the compromise view that both organic and emotional factors are of importance in the aetiology, that both are or can be present in the individual case. Perhaps now it is worth while considering an extension of this compromise view—the possibility that childhood autism is an example of psychosomatic illness with emotional and somatic reactions affecting one another reciprocally, so that circular mechanisms are established.

Ultimately, of course, the deviant behaviour in childhood autism must be the result of abnormal physiological events in the brain. For the child's behaviour is the immediate result of such physiological occurrences. These abnormal physiological occurrences could be due to disease—anatomical, metabolic or ' electrophysiological '—or they could be the attempt by a normal brain to adapt itself defensively against an excessively stressful environment. Perhaps, in a given case, it is not enough to ask whether the factors responsible for the physiological malfunction are anatomical, metabolic or emotional, because there seems no reason why causes from two, or even three, of these groups should not be jointly responsible in any one case.

ORGANIC FACTORS

Constitutional Predisposition

Few psychiatrists nowadays will deny that there must be some predisposition, some organic instability in the brains of those who develop schizophrenic illnesses in childhood or in adult life, and there is compelling evidence, particularly from twin studies, of the importance of genetic factors (Kallman and Roth, 1956; Kay and Roth, 1961). Kallman and Roth studied genetic aspects of pre-adolescent schizophrenia, excluding from their sample ' very young children who presented the clinical picture of a psychosis with mental deficiency, perhaps simulating a severe intellectual defect as the result of a very early schizophrenic process '. This would of course exclude a large proportion of autistic children, and it is uncertain whether their cases included children with physical signs of organic disease of the central nervous system. Their criteria, however, were fairly similar to those later proposed by Dr. Creak and her colleagues (Creak, 1961). Kallman and Roth considered that the inheritance of these schizophrenic children was strikingly similar to that of adult schizophrenics, and suggested that the same genotype (a gene-specific deficiency state) which they assumed to be responsible for the basic symptoms of adult schizophrenia is also present in childhood schizophrenics. They found a definite excess of males over females in the pre-adolescent group, and ' an increase in the number of early schizophrenia cases among the co-twins and sibs of early index cases '. They did not explain why the genotype should produce its effects so very much earlier in some cases than in others, and even if one accepts their genetic findings it appears that one still has to seek non-genetic reasons for the varying age incidence.

Clinically, one is continually impressed by the fact that some children develop psychoses who have been brought up in apparently satisfactory material and emotional environments, without significant physical disease, whereas others, who have been subjected to severe traumata from an early age, nevertheless show little or no sign of psychotic illness. Equally striking, in the writer's present experience, is the fact that he has never seen or heard of a case in which only one of a pair of identical twins is autistic, whereas there have been several cases in which only one of a pair of non-identical twins is autistic, and several more in which both members of an identical twin pair have been autistic or pseudo-autistic (Case No. 14). On the other hand, he has not heard of any case in which both of a non-identical twin pair have been autistic.

Constitutional predisposition is presumably one of the most important factors, not only in causing the illness, but also in determining the time of onset and the type of clinical picture; and this constitutional predisposition must have a physical basis, depending on the inherited genetic structure. It has been suggested that the degree of constitutional predisposition towards schizophrenic reaction must be different in every case, either so slight that only the severest emotional or organic trauma will precipitate schizophrenic breakdown, or, at the other extreme, so strong that minimal traumata can be enough to provoke this kind of deviation. (In this way one could perhaps explain the not infrequent occurrence of cases in which, though the child is described as ' always very backward ' or ' defective from birth ' no neuropathological cause for the condition is found, while the clinical picture shows unmistakable signs of schizophrenia. It seems possible that a number of patients classified as ' congenital mental defect with super-added autism ' may in reality be suffering from ' infantile autism with resultant mental defect '.)

In considering constitutional predisposition, however, perhaps we would be mistaken if we thought exclusively in terms of a specific genetic disease factor or even of a small number of such factors. If we breed racehorses exclusively for speed we are liable eventually to produce an animal whose legs, though they are perfect for sprinting, are nevertheless so delicate, so deficient in adaptive power, that they cannot stand up to racing except under ideal conditions. As soon as the ground gets hard, the horses' legs break down. To take a comparable example in which natural rather than artificial selection produced a similar phenomenon, in prehistory evolution produced enormous creatures which depended for protection from their enemies, and therefore for survival, on their exceedingly heavy armour-plated skin, developed at the expense of adaptability and mobility; in the end the species died out when climatic changes made its excessively heavy integument a liability rather than an asset in the struggle for survival. There are, of course, very many examples of similar over-breeding in nature. The survival and pre-eminence of man has been due largely to his adaptability and to the ability of his brain to react quickly to external stimuli. Through the operation of selective mating highly intelligent men tend to marry women of similar ability, and such mating must be liable to produce children of potentially outstanding intelligence; that is, children with abnormally reactive or 'sensitive' brains. Their brains are like very highly complicated and delicate machines which cannot stand up to rough treatment. Some of these infants might in fact be so sensitive that they were unable to tolerate adverse environmental events which would not seriously disturb an ordinary child. Such a theory might perhaps account for the higher incidence of autism in children whose parents are of superior intelligence (Creak and Ini, 1960).

Another characteristic of man is that the development of the child continues for a very long time after birth. Some animals are fully adult at the moment of birth, and even man's nearest relatives, the anthropoid apes, grow up ten times as quickly as we do. This long period of extra-uterine growth allows for infinitely greater flexibility, with correspondingly higher development of intelligence and ability to respond to training. Instead of fighting his own battles from soon after birth, the human infant has a long period of protection during which he has nothing to do except to develop his body and, in particular, his mind. Delayed maturity seems therefore to be a survival characteristic. Inevitably, however, from time to time, children are going to be born in whom this characteristic is excessively developed, in whom maturity is excessively delayed, and who therefore require very long and favourable periods of complete protection if their potential intelligence is eventually to meet its full realization. Such children might be especially vulnerable and thus driven by unfavourable environmental situations into defence reactions of which the most extreme is, in fact, withdrawal. Perhaps the constitutional predisposition of some children to develop schizophrenic illness could be considered in this light. We might thus account, not only for the fact that the parents of autistic children tend to be of higher intelligence than the general run of the population, but also for the very much higher incidence in boys rather than girls. It is well known that the intelligence of boys tends to be further from the mean than that of girls; also that the human male is, at most ages, more prone to disease, more vulnerable, than the female. On both these counts one would expect boys to be more likely to be affected by the factors mentioned above. These considerations, taken together, may perhaps throw some light on what we mean by constitutional predisposition in autistic children.

Organic Diseases of the Central Nervous System

It has always been commonly believed that the child who is severely defective as the result of physical disease is specially liable to schizophrenic illness, and certainly the schizophrenic syndrome, or something very like it, not uncommonly supervenes in children suffering from, for example, epiloia, phenylketonuria, or brain damage due to anoxia.

Case No. 9. George (born 1.7.54). Admitted to Smiths Hospital 7.6.60
   Summary—Epiloia, with adenoma sebaceum supervening at the age of six and a half years; phenylketonuria; presenting as childhood psychosis but with atypical features preventing diagnosis of childhood schizophrenia; phenylpyruvic acid found in urine;

deterioration in spite of medication with Largactil, Sparine and barbiturates; destructive, hyperkinetic, distractible, heedless, aggressive towards self and others.

Complaint by mother—Can only say ' mama ' and ' dada ' (aged five and a half); tantrums, destructiveness, aggressiveness.

Family—Mother aged 20 at birth of patient, an only child who depends a great deal on her parents. She shows no anxiety about George, no warmth or affection in her reactions to him though she is dutiful and co-operative in a formal way. Father, aged 28 at the child's birth, a bricklayer, quiet but affectionate in relation to George, though showing markedly little anxiety about him. It appeared that both these parents had withdrawn in a self-protective way from the child. One paternal uncle did not speak until four and a half years old. There is no history of mental illness on either side of the family.

History—Mother was depressed during pregnancy and easily upset, though the baby was wanted. Pregnancy otherwise normal, delivery at home, weight $7\frac{1}{2}$ lb. Mother said he was 15 days overdue and born by ' forced labour '. Breast fed for six months. Changed to bottle because milk dried up, and kept on the bottle until age of three. He would then eat solids, but refused to drink any liquid except from a bottle. He sat up at eight months, walked at 18 months, but never learned to say more than ' mama ' and ' dada ' except one or two odd words. Dry by day and night by two and a half years, clean soon afterwards and able to indicate he wanted the pot. General health always good except for bronchitis at the age of two. He had ' convulsions ' from four and a half months to 20 months, infrequently and irregularly. Mother found him cold and unresponsive but contented. He slept for 12 hours a day up to admission. Mother tried to cuddle him but found it difficult because he was unresponsive. He showed no response to speech and was admitted to the Children's Unit at Belmont Hospital from 6.1.58 to 6.7.58. He was described as withdrawn, unco-operative and speechless. He improved only in cleanliness. X-ray showed the right side of the skull was larger than the left, and AEG showed the ventricular system was normal with no obvious thinning of the cortex. EEG showed irregular rhythm in the occipital region on the left side and sharp waves also appeared occasionally in that area. It was suggested that this abnormality might indicate a cortical lesion in the left tempero-occipital region. No abnormal signs were found in the central nervous system. There was no hearing loss. Psychological testing has never been possible. He functions at idiot level. On return from Belmont he was more destructive and hyperkinetic and had difficulty in getting off to sleep.

Mental state—On admission to Smiths Hospital he made no proper rapport with staff, did not take any notice of the children or of the toys and was in fact heedless, treading on or kicking whatever was in his path. He scratched his own face, tore his clothes, was hyperkinetic and speechless. He showed tantrums when thwarted, was clean if potted regularly, also dry, and slept well. He was happiest when put in the baby's pram and wheeled around. He was pathologically preoccupied with a succession of small plastic objects for a few days at a time. Tantrums occurred on attempting to change his rituals. He showed visual avoidance and functioned as if totally deaf. He showed mannerisms, but apart from manual dexterity in manipulating the objects of his choice there were no islands of normal development. He smelled everything in sight, he spent his time jumping up and down, running heedlessly around, or tearing things with his teeth. He ran about a good deal on tip-toe, as in some other brain damaged children showing psychotic features. He fulfilled most of the accepted criteria of childhood schizophrenia. After admission to hospital, phenylketonuria was demonstrated and adenoma subaceum of the face was diagnosed. He has shown slow, steady deterioration and has failed to respond to drugs. He tends to be sleepy on the large doses of Largactil (750 mg. a day) and Sparine (75 mg. a day) he is receiving. Though he does not make relationships with anyone he will respond to a cuddle as one responds to an armchair. His physical health has remained good and he has shown no fits.

There is no reason why schizophrenia should not supervene in a child whose brain has been damaged by trauma, or infectious or metabolic disorder. Indeed, it is possible that a schizophrenic type of reaction might be especially likely to develop in such a child. The vulnerability of these children might, in fact, be due to constitutional predisposition, to their physical disease or injury, or to emotional stress. These then would be regarded as the predisposing factors, working singly or in combination. The precipitating factors might again be physical illness or emotional stress, again working singly or in combination.

The well known work by Heller (1930), Yakolev, Weinberger and Chipman (1948) and Tramer (1935–6) attributes at least some cases of childhood psychosis to ' deteriorating organically determined illness '. Creak (1961) has had similar clinical experiences and quotes cases of the syndrome affecting children who have proved to be suffering from lipoidosis. Certainly, every psychiatrist who works with severely disturbed children will encounter cases of autism or the schizophrenic syndrome who are eventually found to be suffering from deteriorating organic disease of the central nervous system. But although there is such evidence in some cases of the schizophrenic syndrome, in a large proportion there is none. Autistic children seldom die young, so that opportunities for autopsy are rare. Where autopsies have been performed, morbid anatomical lesions have not been found except in those cases which have sickened and died from a generalized disorder such as a lipoidosis (Creak, 1961). For example, one of the present writer's patients, a typical autistic child who slowly became a typical schizophrenic adult, developed typical epileptic fits for the first time at the age of 17 years, and died about a year later in status epilepticus: at autopsy no neurological lesions were found which could be regarded as the cause rather than the result either of his status epilepticus or of his psychosis.

The continuing rude health of most schizophrenic children is another argument against ascribing their condition to an ' organic ' brain pathology; if they had a brain lesion of such severity as to cause complete devastation of the intellect and personality, one would expect them to develop definite neurological physical signs sooner or later; but, in general, they do not. Some authors have described what are called 'soft' physical signs of neurological disease, for example, hypotonia, diminished or absent reflexes, squint and defective co-ordination. But such physical signs, where they have been observed by the present writer, have tended to be inconstant and to fade towards normality as the children grew up. They are, in any case, such as might be observed in otherwise normal children without causing much comment. It would appear, then, that in most cases of childhood autism the chronic neurological lesions, if they exist, are something quite different from any other known kind of neurological pathology. Indeed, it seems questionable whether morbid anatomical lesions are the prime or only cause of symptoms in the majority of cases.

Childhood Autism and Epilepsy

Many autistic children have abnormal electroencephalograms, but those specialists with the greatest experience in this kind of investigation seem to be the least likely to suggest that any particular kind of EEG abnormality is specific for these patients. Indeed, in their reports the words 'non-specific abnormality' occur very frequently. Some of our autistic children do, however, have abnormal EEG's which are more or less typically epileptic, grand mal or petit mal in type; and some patients—not always those with the abnormal EEG's—do have epileptic attacks of various kinds. This has been advanced as favouring an organic aetiology for childhood autism. Certainly, cerebral dysrhythmia must arise ultimately from a physical disturbance in the brain, but it seems worth considering that this disturbance could be caused not only by anatomical lesions in the brain, but also by constitutional instability, by metabolic disorder, or by emotional upset. Inherited constitutional instability might indeed be expected to show itself by EEG abnormality if we knew enough about the EEG.

The ability of some patients to prevent or abort epileptic

fits by an effort of will or by concentrating upon some particular subject, or by some kind of sensory stimulus or motor activity, is well known, as is the ability of some patients to produce typically epileptic attacks on suitable occasions, as, for example, when frustrated, or upon the entrance of the doctor into the ward; and Ounsted (1961) has shown that in some cases, ' fits ' and also the abnormal EEG tracing with which they are associated may be aborted by a sharp command. Idiopathic epilepsy appears to mean epilepsy for which no physical cause is apparent and in which physical changes found in the brain at autopsy are as likely to be the result as the cause of the epileptic attacks. In 1948, Hill pointed out that epileptic attacks can occur in undoubted schizophrenics and suggested that in fact epileptic attacks might be a symptom of schizophrenic illness.

It seems that epilepsy is a symptom and not a disease in its own right, and that factors like constitutional instability in the brain, metabolic disorders, and emotional disturbance, as well as anatomical lesions in the brain, may be important aetiological factors.

Biochemical Disturbances

The work of Gjessing (1938, 1939) showing disturbed nitrogen metabolism in periodic catatonia is, of course, the pioneer work in this field and little further advance occurred until attention was directed towards metabolic aspects of schizophrenia by the success of the tranquillizing drugs. A large number of observations have been made in schizophrenics showing metabolic anomalies, but their significance is far from being understood. Osmond and Smythies (1952) suggested that there was, in schizophrenics, an accumulation of an abnormal methylated compound with hallucinogenic properties, having based their hypothesis on the observation that the hallucinogenic drug mescaline is chemically very similar to methylated compounds found in increased concentrations in the brains of some schizophrenics. Pollin, Cardon and Ketz (1953) found that some chronic schizophrenics who had been maintained on mono-amine-oxydase inhibitors were made temporarily worse by administration of methionine and suggested that this might be due to facilitation, in such patients, of transmethylation of amines. These and similar observations have been confirmed by others, including Brune and Himwich (1963). Friedhoff and van Winkle (1962) detected a substance (which behaves very like 3-4-dimethoxyphenylethylamine) in the urine of a high proportion of schizophrenic patients which was not found in normals. It therefore seems possible that accumulation of one or more methylated compounds plays a significant part in some forms of adult schizophrenia. However, as Quastel and Quastel (1962) observed, ' it has to be clearly understood that whilst alterations in the level of substances such as serotonin and the catecholamines in the brain are affected by the amine oxydase inhibitors, there is no conclusive evidence that these amines are causally involved '. These remarks apply also to the observations mentioned above and to those of Basowitz and his colleagues (1955) on abnormalities in the excretion of hippuric acid after benzoic acid administration in persons under emotional stress, as well as in catatonic schizophrenics and subjects under the influence of mescaline. It also applies to the more recent observations of Hoagland and his colleagues (1962) who claim to have detected a very labile factor in fractions of human globulin which exists in greater quantities in schizophrenics than in normals, and which produces behaviour disturbances in rats. It is of course possible that these metabolic disturbances may be the result of the schizophrenic process rather than its cause.

There have been a few reports of abnormal metabolism in psychotic children (Sutton and Read, 1958; Koegler, Colbert and Eiduson, 1961) but no study of a large series has yet been published, as far as I know. Simon and Gillies (1964) have recently shown that a significant proportion of schizophrenic children have grossly retarded bone age, and that many are also grossly retarded in height and weight. This suggested that there might be some pituitary dysfunction in these cases, and in further investigations Simon has demonstrated impaired glucose tolerance and also impaired insulin tolerance in a significant proportion of autistic children. If Simon's results are confirmed they will constitute fairly conclusive evidence of an abnormality in the pituitary–suprarenal system in a large proportion of these children.

Simon and Gillies (1964) recently suggested that a percentage of hospitalized autistic children show abnormally high concentrations of lead in the blood stream. This work is being confirmed in other quarters (Moncrieff and his colleagues, 1964; Oliver and O'Gorman, 1966) but we do not as yet know whether the high levels of blood lead are due to ingestion of large quantities of lead by normal children who thus become psychotic, or to ingestion of large quantities of lead by children who are already psychotic, and in whom pica is one of the symptoms; or to inability of psychotic children to metabolize lead in the quantities normally available from the diet and environment; or to a combination of two or all of these factors. The analogy of deficient copper metabolism leading to Kinnier Wilson's disease, and the fact that we already know there is a disturbance of metabolism in many of these psychotic children, suggests that the increased blood lead may well be due partly to defective metabolism and not merely to increased ingestion of lead.

Sometimes these indications of endocrine–metabolic disturbance coincide with other observations suggesting endocrine deficiencies in individual cases, for example, the normal infant who suffered from a severe anoxia at the age of 15 months and subsequently underwent psychotic personality change with dwarfism, obesity, raised blood lead, diminished insulin tolerance, severe pica and the replacement of normal hair by a coarse brush of upstanding wiry hair. If it is confirmed that there is, in a high proportion of children suffering from the schizophrenic syndrome, a disturbance of endocrine function

57

involving pituitary, suprarenals, and perhaps the hypothalamus, the thyroid, and the pancreatic islets, then a new series of questions will arise: are we to regard the endocrine disturbance as being primarily in the suprarenal or in the hypothalamus-pituitary? Or is it due primarily to an anatomical lesion of the pituitary, affecting growth and bony development directly and the functioning of the other endocrine glands secondarily? Or is it due to an anatomical lesion in the hypothalamus causing pituitary dysfunction and, through this, dysfunction in the thyroid, the suprarenals and the islets? Or is there an upset in the function of the hypothalamus caused, not by anatomical lesions, but rather by emotional disturbance due to environmental stress? Is the emotional illness (the psychosis) due to upset in function of the pituitary and the other glands, or is it due to dysfunction in the hypothalamus caused by environmental stress? We know that stress can cause physical symptoms which we must presume to be mediated through the hypothalamus, for example, the fainting and dropping blood pressure which can be caused by sudden horror. We know that anxiety can cause an infinite variety of somatic symptoms in which hypothalamic function must be involved. Does it need a great imaginative leap to envisage a chronic disturbance in hypothalamic function, due to emotional factors, which can cause the endocrine dysfunction as well as the withdrawal, the mannerisms, and the other psychiatric symptoms of childhood autism?

In the present state of our knowledge we cannot answer these questions. If lesions could be demonstrated in the pituitary or the other endocrine glands of autistic children, this would be suggestive evidence against a ' psychogenic ' aetiology; but it would not be conclusive, for emotional disturbance might conceivably cause a physical change in the pituitary just as it can cause physical changes in other parts of the body. On the other hand, if a child with psychotic illness and subnormality and emotional disturbance were to show improvement, first as regards his emotional state, later in intellectual functioning, and later still were to show a return to normal endocrine function, this might be evidence in favour of a psychogenic aetiology, but not proof thereof; for it is conceivable that the initial change might have been a marginal improvement in endocrine function. There are children who return to apparent normality following psychotic illness but no follow-up endocrine studies have as yet been reported in such cases.

Delayed Maturation

Bender (1956) and Fish (1960) have suggested that childhood schizophrenia is the result of disturbance or delay in maturation of the central nervous system, and Nouailhat (1960) speaks of irregular or ' anarchic ' patterns of growth in these children. It is true that many autistic children show delayed neurological development, passing the normal milestones in this field much later than normal children, and much later than they pass other milestones of development which should be achieved at about the same time. Bender's views would appear to be supported by the work of Simon, referred to above, which suggests an association in autistic children between endocrine dysfunction and immaturity in certain aspects of development. Daniels (1941) has found that babies under two years of age have much less insulin tolerance than have older children and adults, and this is of interest in view of the impaired insulin tolerance shown by Simon's autistic children. It seems possible that the ' soft ' neurological signs referred to above may also be attributed to relative immaturity in the central nervous system, or in certain parts thereof. Close questioning of a large series of mothers of autistic children shows that only in a minority is there a clear history of normal development. As a rule it emerges that the child was late in talking or lifting his head or appearing to recognize the mother, even though other milestones were passed at normal times. It should be emphasized that these signs of immaturity are not necessarily confined to the central nervous system. There are, for example, a number of autistic children in whom there was delay in development of jaw and pharynx with an associated inability to suck or swallow properly in early infancy. It seems also that prematurity is commoner in a series of autistic children than in the general population, and that, in general, a higher than normal proportion of these children seem to have had difficulty in staying alive in early infancy as the result of intercurrent illness. It would be no surprise if some degree of immaturity were subsequently found in such children.

Case No. 10. Charles. Admitted to Smiths Hospital at age four years eleven months

Summary—Early feeding difficulties with subsequent severe withdrawal; suspected deafness, severe behaviour disorder and retardation.

Mother's description—' Not talking; thumb-sucking continually; about a year behind in everything; rolls himself up in sheets; almost no relationship with people, uses them as tools; preoccupied with machines and water; attached to his own special blanket; little response to danger or pain or sound.'

Family—He is the second of three children; siblings and parents are very intelligent, father a parson and successful headteacher; mother has normally warm relationship with the rest of the family but has not been able to establish a satisfactory relationship with Charles though she is a most co-operative and dutiful parent.

History—Normal pregnancy and birth, 7½ lb. Lower jaw was undeveloped at birth; he could not suck or swallow. He was fed nasally for seven weeks and then spoon fed. He nearly choked with each feed, was terribly distressed and cried when his bib was put on. His mother said ' He got no pleasure from feeding—or from people either—he showed no interest in anything '. He swallowed fluids almost normally by five months and semi-solids by 11 months. At 20 months he swallowed a stone which lodged in his oesophagus. ' Half dead from dehydration ' he was admitted to Great Ormond Street Hospital where he stayed ten days. He was feeding normally by about five years. At three years old he was thought to be deaf and taken to two otologists. No organic hearing loss has ever been demonstrated, indeed his hearing appears to be acute. On 29.5.61 he was admitted to the Radcliffe

Infirmary unconscious, vomiting, with left hemiplegia, extensor planter reflexes, neck stiffness and positive Kernig's sign. EEG showed 'changes consistent with diffuse cerebral abnormality', other investigations were negative. He had a number of generalized convulsions. Burr holes were made showing a rather tense brain. Air ventriculogram showed very small ventricles without any shift or evidence of space occupying lesion. No evidence of encephalitis. General condition improved steadily and after two days he appeared his normal self. There was an epidemic of infective hepatitis at Smiths Hospital at the time but Charles was not jaundiced. He has shown no further fits or neurological signs and his mental state returned exactly to its former state. His EEG on 21.2.62 (sleeping) was regarded as 'probably within normal limits for this age group when asleep'.

Mental state—He has always dribbled and spilt food so that to cuddle him was to get clothes and face smeared with mucous and food residues. He was also liable to bite or poke so that it was not easy to cuddle him. He made only the most fleeting and incomplete contact with children or adults. One could only make a relationship with him through rough or acrobatic play. He sucked his thumb, was preoccupied with surfaces and wheels, and liked spinning objects and twirling ropes. He formed a peculiar relationship with another psychotic child who will allow Charles to take him by the hand and spin him round and round, but otherwise he did not associate. He rarely continued any one activity for more than a minute or so. He ignored most remarks but sometimes obeyed orders and would sit at a table with the others, and could feed himself. He showed normal manual dexterity for anything which interested him. He usually wet the bed.

Electro-physiological Considerations

Perhaps the most important indication that immaturity of the central nervous system is to be found in autistic children lies in the recent work of Grey-Walter (1964). He has developed a new EEG technique by which he has shown that in normal adults required to perform an action in response to a stimulus preceded by a conditional (or warning) stimulus, a negative wave—the 'expectancy wave'—develops in the frontal cortex following the warning stimulus. This negative wave envelops the succeeding electrical responses in the frontal cortex resulting from the second (or imperative) stimulus. The implications of this discovery in electrophysiology must be far reaching, but from the point of view of the present discussion an important feature is that the capacity to develop this expectancy wave response is a measure of the subject's maturity. Mature responses are not universal until the mid-twenties. About half the normal children examined showed mature responses at the age of 15; at seven, mature patterns are beginning to appear in the more precocious or confident children, but the infantile wave form still persists; whilst the corresponding responses in five to eight year olds are variable and show disorderly interactions. In the disturbed children (who were nearly all autistic patients from Smiths Hospital) the pattern of responses was similar to that of much younger normal children. Here, it would appear, is evidence that immaturity in brain development may have something to do with the development of autism in childhood.

It seems legitimate to conclude from all this work (assuming that most of it is confirmed) that even though anatomical lesions of the brain are not very commonly found in autistic children, physiological disturbance can frequently be demonstrated or deduced. The physiological disturbance could be due to genetically determined immaturity, or it could be due to exogenous factors, physical or emotional, or both, acting upon a predisposed child; the predisposition being due to acquired illness, or to genetically determined immaturity, or to a general constitutional predisposition of the kind described above.

EMOTIONAL FACTORS

Even if, ultimately, metabolic or electrophysiological or anatomical pathology is proved in the majority of cases, and a generally applicable pattern of inheritance accepted, it will still be difficult to set aside the weight of opinion, supported by many case histories, which regards emotional traumata as being at any rate important precipitants in producing schizophrenic reactions in childhood (Case Nos. 1 and 3). Those who favour a psychogenic view of the aetiology point to case histories of children suffering from autistic symptoms who, it is claimed, have been improved by psychotherapy and manipulation of the environment, and personal experience of such cases is certainly very striking. At Smiths Hospital it has been found that, although many of the autistic children grow up to become schizophrenic adults, in others considerable improvement has occurred after removal of the child from an incompatible emotional environment at home, with substitute mothering in the hospital, whilst intensive efforts are made to modify family attitudes to the child and his disability, to support and treat the parents in their distress and perplexity, and to improve their methods of handling the child and his symptoms (Case Nos. 1 and 5).

From the clinician's point of view, perhaps the strongest indication that a considerable proportion of cases of childhood autism have a predominantly emotional aetiology lies in the fact that he sees all grades of deviation between the severely deteriorated, completely withdrawn child on the one hand and, on the other hand, the child who is regarded as normal but rather dreamy and remote at times, who has some difficulty in making friends, and who may be described by his mother as tending at times to live ' in a world of his own '. Such children may be completely outgoing and friendly at certain times and with certain people, whereas at other times and with other people they tend to be withdrawn, inert and self-absorbed. They may show a few mannerisms and they may also have a strong tendency towards obsessive rituals or, at least, a paradoxical need for order, or even monotony, in some aspects of their life whilst in others their behaviour is disorganized and at times almost chaotic. When children are brought to the clinic in such a state it is very often possible to modify their condition through psychotherapy—which may sometimes have to be directed as much towards the mother or father as towards the child—and by making alterations in the environmental stresses put upon the child. Thus, a very considerable improvement may be produced, so that the pre-psychotic phase may be merely temporary and not recur. Occasionally, young children, two and three year olds, who are more severely affected in the way of withdrawal and inertia, may make an apparently complete recovery with the same sort of treatment. Of course, there is no reason why a child whose disability is due to organic disease of the brain should not be improved symptomatically by psychotherapy, even though this has no effect on the underlying pathology. We know that such an improvement can be effected in adults suffering from severe anxiety or emotional lability following head injury. But in the children mentioned above we seem to achieve more than symptomatic improvement. Their improvement seems to be due to a halting in the underlying disease process, the child eventually reacting normally, or perhaps neurotically, but not psychotically, in response to environmental stress. In cases like these it is hard to believe that emotional factors have not been important in the aetiology.

Psychodynamic Mechanisms—The Mother-Child Relationship

It seems that in the majority of cases the child's withdrawal from the rest of the environment is really an extension of his initial withdrawal from, or failure ever to make a normal relationship with, his mother. Nearly always there is evidence of impairment at an early stage in the emotional relationship between mother and child, and this is usually associated with some kind of separation, either physical or emotional. Physical separation may be due to illness of one or the other, or to desertion by mother, or even a prolonged holiday away from the child. The illness is frequently described as having begun around the time of the next baby's arrival (Case No. 2) and perhaps this may be explained partly by the temporary separation usual at that time. On the other hand, it may begin during the mother's next pregnancy (Case Nos. 1 and 11). It seems that the mother's relationship to the child may be impaired by her involvement with the new baby, emotionally as well as physically. Emotional separation may be due to inability either of the mother or of the child to make a satisfactory relationship with the other. Sometimes mother is unable to relate adequately because she herself has a schizoid personality (Case Nos. 3 and 7) or she may be suffering from a frank emotional illness; or perhaps she may be clinging to an infantile dependence on her own mother so that she cannot accept the maternal role.

Many writers, including Goldfarb (1961, 1964) have stressed parental inadequacy as being of very great importance in aetiology and have also stressed perplexity on the part of the parents, the perplexity apparently concerning both the parents' role in bringing up children in general, and their methods of dealing with the deviant child. This perplexity on the part of the parents, it is suggested, leads to absence of predictable expectancies in the child with loss of reference and anchoring. Certainly, if the parents' responses are unpredictable, the child must find his relationships with them, and therefore with people in general, more difficult and less rewarding. However, unpredictability in the parents has not been found as a special feature in the present writer's cases, though the preference of the children for things rather than people might be taken as a sign of their distrust of the unpredictability of human beings in general.

Occasionally there is a curious reversal in roles between mother and father, mother being less feminine and more dominant than is usual, and father less masculine and less dominant, so that the child has a satisfactory relationship with neither. Sometimes unhappy relationships between mother and father upset that between mother and child. In other cases, mother seems to be afraid to love the child unreservedly because of father's jealousy.

There have been several instances where the trouble has been associated with early feeding difficulties, the mothers of some of our patients having found breast feeding revolting. In others, the patient has suffered in infancy from severe physical abnormalities like malformations of the jaw which have made early feeding experiences severely traumatic (Case No. 10).

Some of the schizophrenic children have been born prematurely, and seem not to have involved themselves emotionally in a world on which their original physical hold has been precarious. Severe illness in early infancy may have a similar effect. If delayed growth patterns are shown to be a cause rather than a result of the illness, it is possible that such neurological immaturity might act in the same way as premature birth, rendering the child incapable of making an emotional relationship in the early days. The same effect might be caused through sheer physical malformation—it would, as an extreme example, not be expected that an anencephalic monster would be capable of making an emotional relationship. This may be one of the causes of the frequency of the schizophrenic syndrome in severely subnormal children. There seems, in fact, to be no end to the number and variety of factors which may be associated with the breakdown of relationship between these children and their mothers. But such a breakdown is in fact one of the commonest features of the disease (Kaplan, 1950; Winnicott, 1953).

If the child cannot relate to the mother she gets no response, no ' feed back ' in her efforts to love him, and again a vicious circle is set up. In fact it appears that the withdrawal is in a sense mutual. The more mother detaches herself from the baby the more he withdraws from her. The more he withdraws the less lovable he is. Many of these children, by the time they are referred to us, seem quite unlovable, mostly because they cannot themselves relate to another human being, but also because there is no apparent spark of interest or intelligence except in the way they manipulate their familiar objects. Often, moreover, the child shows what seems to be an active refusal to participate in mother's world, a refusal which many parents find intolerable. It is extremely difficult for a mother to continue to love unreservedly a child who disgraces her every time she takes him into the town, who destroys any loose objects of furniture in the home, who keeps her awake half the night, or who seems to be forever trying to dash headlong out of the garden and into the road. In spite of the fact that mother has the child all day while father is out at work, it is father's patience that wears thin most quickly in the majority of cases and it is he, usually, who begins to find the child, and his effect upon the home, intolerable. Quarrels develop between the parents and the brothers and sisters (who are, of course, unable to invite their friends into the house), and, as the child grows older, family life becomes almost impossible. Sometimes the child is unlovable for physical reasons; he may be always covered in excretions of various sorts, for example (Case No. 10); or perhaps he smells; or perhaps, in his heedless mannerisms, he is liable to hurt people.

If this first relationship with his mother fails, then one would expect the child to have difficulty in forming satisfactory relationships with other people. Human relationships will tend to be unrewarding and unsatisfying to him and he will not make them. This has a vitally important effect upon the child's intellectual development, for observation of normal children suggests that their interest in reality as a whole is derived from their interest in people—from their emotional relationships. The child will only want to be part of, or progress in, mother's world if he is sufficiently identified emotionally with her. If he cannot relate normally to his mother, then he must find an adequate mother substitute; for, unless a satisfying love relationship can be formed with some human being, the child may either fail to involve himself to a normal extent in reality or, if he is already involved, he may withdraw.

Partial Withdrawal

Failure of the relationship with mother or mother substitute is, of course, rarely complete. The child will nearly always make some kind of emotional relationship in his earliest days, and will have some degree of involvement with his environment. But in few of our patients is there a completely normal early history in this respect. The child is often described as having been too good, or too quiet, as a baby, as having been slow to respond to his mother or to smile, as having made no co-operative movement when about to be picked up. Usually, some or many of the milestones are delayed, but the mother may think there is nothing wrong, or she may be erroneously reassured, and believe she merely has a sleepy placid baby. In some cases, on the other hand, the milestones may be passed normally or even precociously, the withdrawal beginning later, insidiously or, in some patients, quite rapidly. But in either case the withdrawal or non-involvement is rarely complete, even at the most severe stages. The child takes some interest in somebody or something, even if the interest seems defective or perverted. His interests in reality will probably be on an extremely primitive level—interest in food, or in sunshine and shadow, or the texture of surfaces, or the little noises of leaves, or the lavatory flush. He may come for a cuddle, or show that he wants the pot, or sit up quietly at the table at mealtimes. Always, however, his involvement with people, and their conventions, and their teachings, and their chattels, is qualified; or we can express the situation differently by saying his withdrawal is *partial*.

If early relationships with people have been unsatisfying rather than intolerable—unsatisfying because they have been insufficiently rewarding, or sustained, or reliable—the child may tend to regard new relationships with suspicion and enter into them incompletely or superficially, so that he is partially withdrawn. In this way he would protect himself against further frustration.

The depressive condition suffered by temporarily deprived children has been very clearly described (Bowlby, 1951) and is well recognized. But there is, in most cases of depression in childhood, an element of withdrawal. Presumably the degree of withdrawal must depend largely on the child's inherited constitution, though sometimes the situation to which the child may be exposed is so traumatic that it seems he can only protect himself by a temporary or partial withdrawal. In these cases, the condition nearly always clears up when the life situation again becomes tolerable. But a child in whom the reaction pattern of withdrawal has become established will tend the more easily to resort to this defence whenever the environment becomes especially threatening or frustrating, and once the habit of withdrawal has become established it is hard indeed to break.

Often the mother of a schizophrenic child will protest that the patient is not withdrawn, that he does have a relationship with her although he does not interest himself in other children, or in adults, or in speaking or reading, or generally in making progress. Some of these cases may be examples of the ' symbiotic ' relationship described by Mahler (1952) in which the child permits a relationship based on physical dependence which might almost be regarded as an attempt to return as nearly as possible to the womb. Such a child will be disinclined to make any more mature relationship with his mother, or any relationship at all with another person.

Sometimes the child may appear to be in normal rapport with his mother or with other children around him, but if anyone attempts to increase the degree of intimacy in the relationship, or to intrude further than having a mere tomboy romp, for example, or to persuade the child to learn or to listen, he will protect himself from such further intrusion by running away or by shutting off his attention—in a word, by increasing the degree of his withdrawal for the time being

(Case No. 11). Some of our patients have occasioned controversy because, so far from failing to make personal relationships, they make facile contact with every person (or rather, every adult) whom they meet. They seem to enjoy physical contact with these adults and are fond of such gestures as kissing and stroking (Case No. 7). Yet at no time do such children form a normal relationship with other children, and their relationship with adults is on a purely superficial level. The adult feels no warmth towards the child, no more warmth than he experiences in his relationships with another autistic child who may be mute and inaccessible. If severe pressure is put on such a child he may react by becoming more obviously withdrawn or by other defensive mechanisms like running away, an increase in obsessional preoccupations, or psychosomatic symptoms. Perhaps, in Christine's case (No. 7), the epileptic attacks she produced when under pressure could be regarded as such a defence mechanism. This ability to make only superficial personal relationships is, of course, also found in persons who are not regarded as psychotic or severely disturbed. It is another aspect of this widespread mechanism of partial withdrawal.

Selective Withdrawal

Sometimes the withdrawal is from one whole field of experience or activity, the child permitting himself to take part in other fields of development or activity to a greater or lesser extent. He may show *selective mutism*, speaking to only one or two people, or perhaps to nobody, although he will join in songs or speak quietly into the bedclothes at night when he thinks no-one is listening; or he may show *selective deafness*, hearing perfectly in some situations but not at all, apparently, in others. He may show *visual avoidance*, looking only at what interests him; or he may withdraw from the whole field of *learning*, showing complete disinclination to use his intelligence except in pursuance of his mannerisms or his current preoccupations.

It is of course obvious that the phenomena of partial withdrawal and selective withdrawal are not to be seen only in children diagnosed autistic. There are normal children who hear invitations but not prohibitions; who are ' good at French but hopeless at Latin '; who can only be taught by certain teachers, and can never learn anything from a parent; who cannot see the article they have been sent upstairs to fetch. Surely some at least of these children are thus limited through *emotional* factors, and are in fact ' selectively withdrawn '.

There are, moreover, very many children who are partially withdrawn from human relationships, or indeed from reality as a whole, either temporarily or as a permanent feature of their personalities. If such partial withdrawal persists, the process may eventually result in the cold ' schizoid ' personality who finds difficulty in making close friends. If the process is continued in later childhood and accentuated and, in particular, if the child is treated cruelly, he may become one of those affectionless psychopaths who are liable to become irreclaimable delinquents. There may in fact be a continuum between normality, on the one hand, through the reserved suspicious individual, the cold, mildly schizoid personality, the schizoid psychopath, and the withdrawn autistic youth, to the florid juvenile schizophrenic on the other.

These concepts, of partial withdrawal and selective withdrawal, and of the continuum between normality and severe schizophrenia, might have some application in fields beyond the present study. At any rate, they seem to have some relevance in accounting for symptoms of childhood autism and further reference will be made to them in subsequent pages.

CHAPTER 5

THE SYMPTOMS OF AUTISM

FAILURE TO SPEAK

Loss of, or failure to acquire, speech is one of the most characteristic features of the severely autistic child. It is of course not pathognomonic of the condition, but it is one of its commonest features. The classical story is of the child who learned to say a few words or was talking almost normally at the age of two and a half and whose speech then stopped improving, the child talking less and less until in the end only a few words or none at all were left. Many of the children thus affected obviously understand everything that is said to them, and one knows they could talk perfectly well if they wished to; indeed, from time to time when they are away from interested adults, or when there is no pressure on them, they may come out with perfectly apposite sentences, and then relapse into silence for months or even years. Just occasionally they may be provoked into making a remark by some sudden emotional crisis; or they may retain one word as a means of keeping the world away—usually ' no '. Several of our patients talk to themselves in their cots at night, or join in songs, or utter odd inappropriate sentences, but they will not use speech for communication (Case Nos. 3 and 11). Most interesting of all is the way in which mute schizophrenic children learn to speak in those cases which improve under treatment. The child does not learn in monosyllables like ' mama ' and ' dada ' and ' car ', but will remain mute until his emotional state has reached a point at which he is ready to resume speech. He will then begin by repeating a whole phrase or sentence, the organization of which is commensurate with the general intellectual level at which he is functioning (Case Nos. 3, 8 and 11).

PLATE I

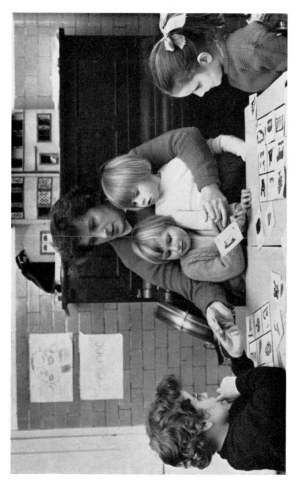

All four children are emerging from severe withdrawal, and beginning to respond to teacher's efforts to get them to tolerate the group in a shared interest.

PLATE II

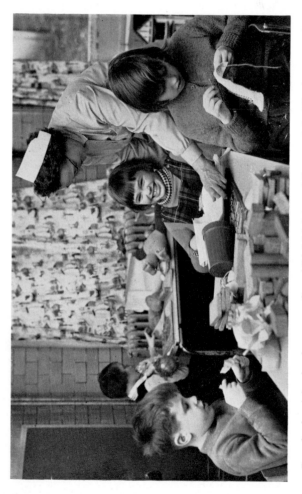

Pre-school training by the nurse. One child (right) is usefully occupied. The boy can only give fleeting attention to the task in hand. The girl in the background has her right hand and arm full of toys from which she refuses to be separated, her mouth full of small objects. But she is doing a little with her left hand, and this is a beginning. The girl in the middle laughs loudly, but refuses to try.

PLATE III

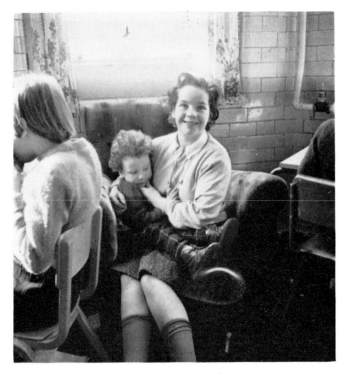

The adolescent girl makes only the most superficial relationships. There is no real warmth between her and the autistic child she is cuddling.

PLATE IV

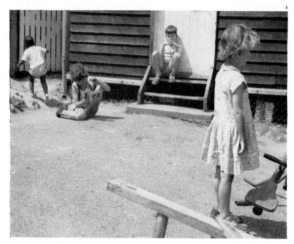

Together, but alone; and unoccupied except in mannerisms.

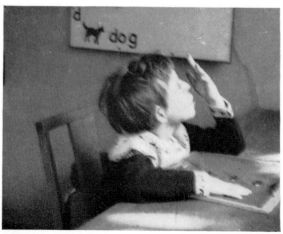

Mannerisms interfere with attempts at occupation and
training.

PLATE V

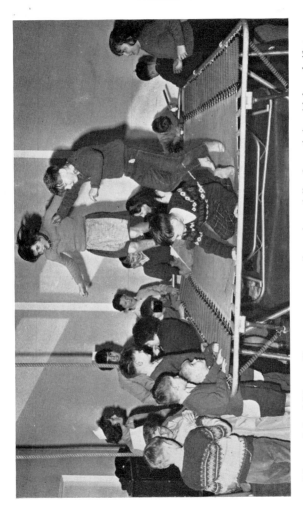

Most autistic children will emerge, temporarily and partially, from their withdrawal, if an intensely exciting atmosphere can be produced. The trampoline was new and all but a few responded to the excitement of a new and boisterous physical activity.

PLATE VI

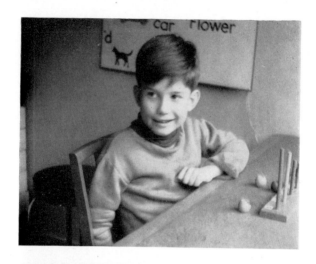

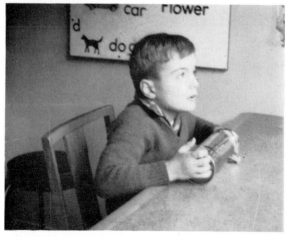

Two boys who resist attempts to occupy them—one holds the toy but stares vacantly ahead; the other turns aside with his perpetual smile.

PLATE VII

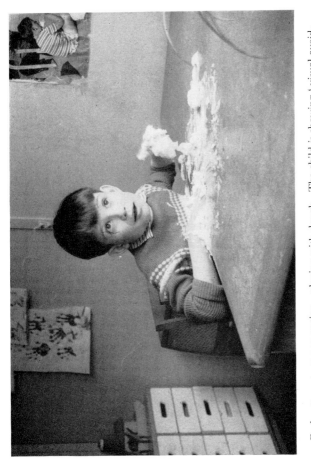

Early attempts at occupation—playing with dough. The child is showing 'visual avoidance'—failing to look at photographer or camera or dough.

PLATE VIII

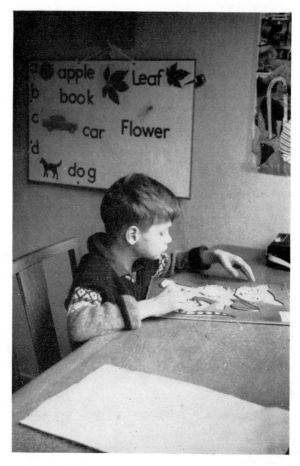

The boy who was tube-fed every day of his life until
coming to the hospital at the age of five, and held his
head up only briefly. His jaw and his neck muscles have
still not developed normally.

The schizophrenic child, when he does speak, often adopts a peculiar tone, and his speech may be nasal and monotonous. Sometimes he speaks like an organically deaf child, even though no organic cause for the deafness can be found (Case No. 12) and the child in fact hears very well. Neologisms, baby babble and playing inappropriately with single words or sentences are all common. Just as these children are willing to use their muscles in aimless, though often complicated activity, unrelated to the real world (and thus differing from a normal child's play) so they will use their faculty of speech aimlessly, as an exercise unconnected with the normal communicative purpose of speech (Adams and Glasner, 1954). Such children might be described as withdrawn from the field of communication. If this were the only aspect of reality from which the child is withdrawn, he would be diagnosed as a case of selective mutism but probably not as autistic; in fact, the condition would be more likely to be regarded as a kind of hysteria. As a rule, however, a selectively or generally mute child shows a number of other autistic features.

FAILURE TO HEAR

A related phenomenon is psychotic deafness. Most schizophrenic children are accused, at some time or other, of being deaf. In several cases of children considered totally deaf, careful audiological examination has made it doubtful whether there is in fact any severe organic hearing loss (Case No. 11). Here again the failure to hear, or rather the failure to respond to auditory stimuli, is part of the child's withdrawal. He is withdrawn from that aspect of reality, among others, which has to do with sound or, at any rate, with speech. Like mutism, the deafness is often selective, that is, towards certain individuals only; or it may involve only the spoken word; or it may be total (and of a severity which is very rarely seen in the organically deaf child); or, most confusing of all, it may at times be an exact imitation of partial nerve deafness, or high tone deafness, or word deafness. This kind of hearing difficulty is, of course, very similar to the functional or hysterical deafness found in certain neurotic adults.

The problem of the deaf and non-communicating psychotic child brings in one of the most controversial questions in regard to the symptomatology of schizophrenic children, namely: ' If a child undergoes functional hearing loss during the age period at which the essential neurological organization of speech function ought to be going on, to what extent is it possible for the child to carry out this organization and learning at a later stage when the cerebral plasticity essential for the learning process has been lost? ' We know there are certain skills which can only be learned in childhood; for example, it is hard for a child to learn to use his auditory or his speaking functions properly if he has not begun to do so at the appropriate age. This would account for the extreme difficulty we have in teaching the schizophrenic child to speak if he is still mute at the age of five years, even though we have been able to produce an apparently substantial improvement in his emotional state. It might also account for the fact that, when the occasional non-communicating psychotic child who improves under treatment begins to speak, his speech may be very like that of an organically deaf child (Case No. 12).

When a child who has no discernible disease of the ear or the auditory nerve and no history of trauma or infection to explain his disability, but nevertheless fails to respond to, or shows an apparent inability to comprehend the spoken word, he has in the past been diagnosed as suffering from ' auditory aphasia ', or, more accurately, ' auditory agnosia '. It has been supposed that this condition is due to congenital organic disease in the auditory area or speech area, so called, of the cerebral cortex. Demonstration of such pathology at autopsy must be excessively rare—the present writer has been unable to find an authenticated case—but prolonged clinical observation of a number of children diagnosed as aphasics has suggested that, in them, emotional disturbance is very common; indeed, a considerable proportion of them can be confidently regarded as autistic. It seems legitimate to wonder whether a good many ' auditory aphasics ' are in reality ' chronic non-listeners '.

It is hard to imagine what anatomical lesion or endocrine disturbance could explain the behaviour of a child who hears some people but is deaf to others with voices of similar tone; or who responds to quiet sounds at the beginning of an audiological test session but fails to respond later or in subsequent tests. What lesion could be the cause of a child's failing to speak for a very long period, then making an entirely appropriate remark under emotional stress, then relapsing into silence again for a further long period? The case of Ellen is an example.

Case No. 11. Ellen. Admitted to Smiths Hospital aged two and a half years

Summary—Delayed walking; no response to sound but presence of good hearing demonstrated; failure to speak or to learn although she shows intelligent normal play; panics, followed by withdrawal, if environment becomes threatening or coercive.

Complaint by mother—Does not speak or seem to hear; can climb but will not walk; temper tantrums; ' won't do anything for me '.

Family—She has one brother two years older and one three years younger. There was a still-born daughter 18 months after Ellen's birth. There was no abnormal family history.

History—Pregnancy—vomiting early, haemorrhages later, for which mother was confined to bed at seven months and induced at eight months. No physical abnormalities at birth but Ellen was very quiet and passive. Breast feeding was discontinued after two weeks due to insufficient milk. Weaning was commenced at seven to eight months but was unsuccessful, that is to say, Ellen's appetite was very poor and she refused all solids and would only take fluids from the bottle right up to the time of admission, aged two and a half years. She lifted her head at 12 months, sat up at 18 months and crawled soon afterwards. She stood alone at two years and climbed about the furniture and out of her cot, upon which mother put a lid, but could not walk on admission. She never spoke or responded to the spoken word. She refused toilet

training completely. At 18 months she was referred to a paediatrician who described her as grossly backward; but at two years
he described her as ' extremely active, crawls frantically about and
gets about on her feet but is always falling '. Seen when aged two
years three months by the writer she evidently had normal co-
ordination and power in her limbs; yet, though she would crawl
about on the furniture, she did not walk more than a step or two
without falling. She did not speak or respond to sound. She
responded to cuddling by her parents but ignored her elder
sibling. Her manner was bright and alert but she did not respond
to people except through cuddling or romping. If mother tried to
feed her with a spoon or cup, Ellen let her lower jaw fall so that the
fluid dribbled out. She had one petit mal attack at two years and
one grand mal at five and a half years.

Mental state—On admission she was restless and over active,
smiled at everyone and did not seem to notice the parents' departure. Within 24 hours she was walking—though she still fell quite
a lot—using the pot, feeding with spoon and cup, including solids,
and sleeping normally in a bed. Her social competence improved
steadily after admission and at six and a half she played normal
imaginative games with the other children. With adults she was
affectionate on the surface and mischievous, but her relationships
were entirely superficial and based mostly on games and physical
contact. If any pressure was put on her she might show panic in
the form of a tantrum and, if pressure were continued, she would
withdraw, running away or making no response. She was untestable until she was 4 : 8 years old, when the psychologist
gave her a mental age on the Merrill Palmer test of two and a
half years. In 1962, at the age of 6 : 3 her mental age on the
same test was 6 : 3, the psychologist concluding that her intelligence is probably within the average range. She continued to
ignore auditory stimuli, although special testing at the Reading
Audiological Unit, and the use of EEG techniques, indicated that
she had adequate and perhaps normal hearing. She did not speak
except for odd words, nearly always when she believed she was
unobserved, and on one occasion when Matron returned from a
long absence she said, in great excitement, ' Look, it's Matron '.
Reports of her using isolated words and phrases, perfectly
enunciated, came from neighbours as well as from the staff at the

hospital. In school she joined in the games but made no effort at all to learn or to lip read. If pressed, she withdrew.

She posed a dilemma: should we continue to treat her psychosis and attempt to persuade her to hear and speak and learn, or should we treat her as a deaf child and try to teach her by methods used ordinarily with deaf children? In the end we decided to treat her as deaf, but the response to education was much less than would have been expected from a child with her intelligence quotient, even if severely deaf. She violently and consistently resisted wearing a deaf aid. In school she showed only very limited application and resisted instruction, tending to 'shut off' and withdraw attention when pressure was applied.

Was there a basic anatomical lesion in Ellen which caused a failure to respond to sound or to speak, other than on rare occasions? If so, was there another anatomical lesion which prevented her from walking but enabled her to climb about the furniture? Was there a third lesion which prevented her from opening her mouth or swallowing when fed with a spoon whilst allowing her to open her mouth and suck normally from a bottle—and to feed herself normally within a few hours of admission to hospital? It is, of course, commonplace that adults rendered aphasic by a cerebral catastrophe may sometimes speak in moments of stress, but it is difficult to imagine that a comparable pathology could exist in Ellen. At the age of nine Ellen is moving normally, showing some progress in school, but functioning as a deaf child and making the kind of noises one hears from a severely deaf child aged four or five. Perhaps Ellen did have, and does have, a number of very tiny lesions in different parts of her brain which cause these symptoms, but the suggestion that they are due to a prolonged selective withdrawal does seem a reasonable alternative. Is it possible that, just as a severely frightened adult may be found hysterically deaf, so Ellen, for her own emotional reasons, became hysterically deaf; or to express it differently, that she withdrew from sound in early childhood? If, for emotional reasons, sounds were excluded at this stage—when she would

77

normally have been learning to appreciate sound and to speak —might it be possible that the neurological development essential to the process of hearing and speaking did not take place, rendering her for practical purposes deaf and dumb? In other words, is it possible that emotional factors operating during the phase of development can have caused a failure of physiological or even anatomical differentiation which could prevent the acquiring of normal function?

One of the most interesting features about Ellen is that there is complete disagreement among those who know her best as to whether she is truly deaf and dumb. Her parents, with whom she has for a long time spent every week-end, now tend to the belief that she is deaf, but they say that several neighbours claim to have heard her speak. The teachers in the hospital school also feel that she must be organically deaf and dumb, though the head teacher, who has very wide experience with deaf children, wonders why she is so resistant to wearing her hearing aid. All the staff wonder why a child who is so bright and sensible in other ways, and who plays so normally, should make so little response to attempts at intensive teaching. In the schoolroom she functions as deaf and dumb and mentally subnormal. Outside school she functions as deaf and dumb, but in her play she is very like a normal child. The Matron of the hospital, who has enormous experience and who has known Ellen intimately since she was an infant, has never had any doubt that Ellen can hear and speak. Her audiological tests have been carried out by Dr. Kevin Murphy, who has unrivalled experience in this field and with this type of child. He has found that Ellen's response to auditory stimuli has been inconsistent. At the first testing session he noted that Ellen responded to some sounds, and that she responded, in his view unmistakeably, to the *withdrawal* of very quiet sounds. In subsequent tests she has shown much less response to auditory stimuli.

The present writer, who knows Ellen well but has never achieved great intimacy with her, has never been able to trap her into an unequivocal response to auditory stimulus, but can add one observation about her which may be of interest: Ellen has never been totally or generally withdrawn; she was somewhat hyperkinetic as an infant but this tendency has diminished. She does make emotional relationships, but these do not seem to be on as deep a level as those seen in most children, though in this respect she has come nearer to normality as the years have passed. But if pressure is put on Ellen to get her to make some intellectual effort, or to get her to respond to instructions given by speech and by mime, she becomes increasingly unresponsive. If the pressure is continued she will attempt to run away, and if she is prevented from running away she becomes seriously withdrawn and remains so until the situation is terminated.

Finally there is Ellen's response to attempts to get her to lip read, which is nil. The two special teachers of the deaf who have experience of Ellen explain this by recalling that ' some children just cannot lip read '. Presumably, organic lesions which would prevent her from hearing and speaking and functioning at a normal level intellectually would also make it very difficult for her to lip read, but in Ellen's case the situation is not quite so simple; for Ellen will not even look at one's lips when one tries to get her to lip read. She looks away, in any direction but at one's lips, showing typical visual avoidance. If one presses to make her look at one's lips her expression becomes glassy and for the time being she is unmistakeably withdrawn.

Possibly an even more instructive case than Ellen's is that of Freddie.

Case No. 12. Freddie. Admitted to Smiths Hospital aged four years eight months

Parents' complaints—Mischievous; over active; aggressive; has tantrums; will not settle to sleep.

History—He was born at full term and weighed 5 lb. 2 oz. There were no difficulties at labour nor was there any neonatal illness.

His mother was 21 at the birth. In pregnancy she had rubella at 13 weeks, dysentery at six months. She was sick, depressed and inert, especially during the first three months, and she had frightening dreams about the baby. These persisted for two years after the birth. The domestic circumstances during Freddie's first two years were disturbed and difficult. There were serious problems of accommodation and a good deal of family strife. His mother does not remember being especially depressed after the birth, but she has continued to have recurrent periods of depression, and these bouts are accompanied by nightmares. Her emotional state has been much affected by her husband with whom her relationships have been very poor throughout. The father seems frequently to have been emotionally disturbed and has recently been in a mental hospital for several months. He has been variously diagnosed as suffering from alcoholism, depression and psychopathic personality. The parents eventually separated.

Freddie was a difficult baby from birth. His mother could not breast feed and said she had to ' fight ' him to get him to take the bottle. He remained very difficult and faddy over food until admission. As a baby he screamed very much, day and night. He walked at 12 months and was clean and dry at three and a half years.

His first words, apart from ' mama ' at about nine months were ' pick it up ' at 14 months, this phrase being associated with the game of throwing objects on to the floor from his perambulator. He learned no more words for a further 18 months. Just before his second birthday he was seen by a ' specialist ' who told mother he was deaf. His mother said his hearing always seemed very variable, but that at times he did not respond even to loud speech. By the age of four and a half years he was exceedingly aggressive towards his brother and sister, had tantrums when crossed in any way, and his mother stated he was completely unmanageable.

On admission to hospital he calmed down a good deal and fed normally. He has always been extremely difficult to manage in the hospital and on holidays with his parents he behaved very badly. Two attempts to get him into the local primary school failed because of his uncontrollable behaviour. At first he mostly used only single words but he could use phrases like ' Freddie's poorly now '. His speech has continued to be very poorly articulated, resembling in some ways that of a severely deaf child. Hearing has varied very greatly. At times he has responded to the quietest sounds, at others only to the very loudest. Usually he appears to hear better if he can see the examiner's lips, but often he has indisputably responded to quiet sounds made well out of his vision. When he was six years ten months, the audiologist reported, ' It is quite possible that he has a loss of perhaps 30 decibels. However, he must be hearing down to this level with at least one ear'. (This level of hearing ought to be enough at least to enable the child to speak almost normally and to respond to classroom teaching, especially if the sound is amplified. Freddie did seem to respond better when he was wearing a hearing aid, but showed a considerable reluctance at most times to wear it.) Four months later the audiologist reported, ' I am convinced he is not deaf'. The ophthalmologist reported, '. . . scattered pigmentation in both fundi. Vision 6/12ths. Looks like abiotrophy.' This latter finding is, of course, extremely important in view of the history of maternal rubella, although the mother did not have this illness until the 13th week of pregnancy so that the effect of this disease as regards development of his auditory and visual apparatus may not have been important.

At the age of seven years, special electroencephalographic examination by Dr. Grey-Walter showed that his ' non-specific responses to visual stimuli were large, slow, prolonged and extensive. Those to auditory stimuli were similar but smaller. There was little habituation but marked contingent occlusion of auditory by visual responses. The pulse rate was high (110) throughout and rose to 140 on presentation of the first auditory stimuli. The mean respiration rate was 25 with brief acceleration to 70 for the first presentation. The psychogalvanic responses were abundant and clearly grouped into short (1·5 sec.) and long (1·8 sec.) latency populations'. The EEG showed no features which could be regarded as abnormal in a child of that age, and indeed all the routine EEG examinations have shown no definite abnormality, except that on one occasion the record was considered to show some features which are sometimes seen in temporal lobe epilepsy. No attacks of epileptic type disturbance have been observed clinically.

Freddie has a full range of speech sounds, which strongly indicates that he has adequate hearing for speech. All the hospital staff, as well as his parents, agree that at times he appears to hear well, and some have likened the variability of his hearing to the variability of squint in other children. At school he is about two years retarded and his backwardness and failure to learn are in marked contrast to his generally intelligent play. Estimates of his I.Q. have varied considerably. If performance items alone were used he scored at times 10 or 20 points below the average for his age, at other times several points above the average. He scored very poorly on verbal items and this was attributed by the psychologists to his having failed to understand instructions.

Freddie is not generally withdrawn, he plays normally though aggressively. He could not be described as an autistic child, though he has been very severely disturbed. Upon short acquaintance with him, teachers and nurses have tended to attribute his aggressiveness to frustration at inability to hear and speak properly, but nearly everyone who has known him for several years finds it difficult to resist the impression that his frequent failure to respond to sound may be associated with a failure to listen or attend, or to an intermittent and partial withdrawal from, or dissociation of, the speech function.

Freddie, then, was never seriously withdrawn in the matter of relationships, though he too had this same superficial relationship with most people that has been described in Ellen's case (No. 11). He, too, functioned as severely deaf and spoke like a severely deaf infant. He was exceedingly hyperkinetic and impossibly aggressive. In his family home he becomes increasingly unbiddable and aggressive and has to be returned to the hospital. However, he has made a very slow but, by now, a marked improvement. His speech and hearing have improved slowly and steadily. Now he functions as an only slightly deaf child. He responds to attempts to make him speak or hear, not by withdrawal, but by trying to run away and by reverting to aggressive and unco-operative behaviour. It would appear that Freddie's difficulties with speech and hearing cannot be due to a progressive neurological lesion or collection of lesions. They could be due to relative immaturity of part of his brain due to delayed development in that area, with an emotional reaction to his frustration at being unable to communicate; or they could be due to an emotional disturbance in early childhood which caused the same sort of withdrawal from the hearing and speech function which was postulated in Ellen's case. This kind of withdrawal might be regarded as very similar to what would in the adult be called hysterical aphasia and hysterical deafness.

Cases like those of Ellen and Freddie become even more instructive when considered along with those of many other patients who begin to learn to speak normally at about the normal time or after only slight or moderate delay, but who then lose their speech and at the same time become progressively less responsive to the spoken word though they are rarely found to be functioning as deaf on audiological testing; and with others who are dumb all day but speak or sing the words of songs to themselves when they are alone in their cots at night. One child learned to speak with only moderate delay but then progressively lost his speech and now functions as completely dumb though he can obviously hear very well. He had also learned to draw very well for his age; but now he will do little except cover the paper with an endless succession of curving lines. In this case there was much resistance from the parents to the suggestion that he should be admitted to Smiths Hospital and he became increasingly withdrawn in the extremely distressed family situation which obtained. Finally he was admitted to hospital, but at a stage at which one doubted very much whether much improvement could be achieved, and he has remained almost static since admission. This is, of course, a severely autistic child.

No matter whether the child's hearing difficulties are due to true deafness or to aphasia or to selective withdrawal, we might expect that in consequence of them the cerebral organization needed to cope with what is heard, and to relate it to speech and other mental activity, might not have developed at the proper time; this defect being more severe in the aphasics because of neurological damage, and in the non-listeners because such children might have a disinclination to think as well as to listen. Indeed, we wonder whether a child who has never listened properly to the spoken word might eventually become truly unable to hear in the accepted meaning of the word, just as even a normal adult who is suddenly enabled to see for the first time in his life has difficulty in making use of what he sees and in fitting visual symbols into the pattern of his mental activity.

VISUAL AVOIDANCE

Whereas most autistic children are accused at some time or other of being deaf, and whereas a very high proportion of them either do not speak at all or have severe impairment of speech, one rarely encounters autistic children who are 'functionally' blind. For a long time this seemed to constitute an objection to the general theory of autistic withdrawal as a cause of sensory impairment in children in whom organic lesions could not be demonstrated.

It is evident that in a large proportion at least of autistic children, the apparent deafness is due to auditory avoidance or failure to listen. Such children also tend to show the phenomenon of visual avoidance, of which Ellen's refusal to look at the lips of the person speaking to her may be regarded as an example. Often, autistic children will not look straight at the person who is speaking to them; they look away from him or look beside him or they look 'through' him. Sometimes they just close their eyes, and this may give a clue as to why visual avoidance has been less commented upon than the apparent deafness of autistic children. The essential fact is that human beings do not have earlids. Moreover, they do not have functioning muscles of the external ear, nor do their ears have anything comparable to the iris by which the eye can limit the amount of light reaching the retina. Unwelcome sights can be excluded by turning the head; unwelcome sounds cannot. How then is the child to protect himself from excessive noise or from unwelcome sounds? He can diminish the tension on the ear drum and the stapes by relaxing the tensor tympani and stapedius muscles in the middle ear, but the protection thus afforded is very limited. Presumably the protective mechanism

84

is a central one, either in the inner ear or in the cochlear nucleus or eslewhere in the brain stem, or at a higher level in the brain. If we turn again to the work of Grey-Walter quoted on p. 81, we find a pertinent observation, ' In the *disturbed children*, non-specific responses to visual stimuli were completely absent in four and to auditory stimuli in nine; in most of these, however, there were autonomic responses to the various stimuli. In three disturbed children and one older delinquent there were interactive non-specific responses but no autonomic responses.' In the disturbed children, then (most of whom were autistic children from Smiths Hospital), there were nine children in whom there was evidence that the auditory stimulus had reached the hypothalamus (otherwise the autonomic responses elsewhere in the body would presumably not have occurred) but the non-specific responses were not being observed in the EEG taken from the frontal cortex. The stimulus was reaching the hypothalamus but was not reaching the frontal cortex. In four children the visual stimuli were reaching the hypothalamus (and causing autonomic responses) but not reaching the frontal cortex. Somewhere between hypothalamus and frontal cortex these stimuli were being shut off or dissociated. It seems reasonable to suppose that this may be the mechanism by which the child protects itself from excessive or unwanted stimuli, particularly auditory stimuli.

Other recent researches have shown that the human infant has at a very early stage a propensity for fixing his gaze upon the eyes of his attendant, usually the mother. Even if the mother wears a mask he will fix his eyes upon hers, and even if he is presented with a picture of a face in which the eyes stand out as definite features although the rest of the fact is poorly delineated, the baby will fix his gaze upon the eyes of the picture. Evidently, then, this propensity for gazing upon the eyes of the mother is a vitally important stage in the development of the child. It seems, in fact, to be one of the very first stages in the development of the emotional tie between mother and child.

If for some reason the child did not thus look at the mother's eyes, then one would expect that he would be severely handicapped in making the initial relationship with his mother upon which intellectual as well as emotional development may in large measure depend. Among the reasons for such a failure to look at the mother's eyes might be delayed maturity, or birth injury to the occipital cortex, or absence of any one to look at, or a disinclination of the mother to look at the child, or some kind of physical or emotional disturbance in the child.

A recent case reported by Dr. Cyril Williams (1966) is that of a child who failed to look at the mother's eyes at any stage, nor indeed, would she fixate any object towards which her mother tried to get her to direct her gaze. At first she was thought to be blind, but subsequent investigations and everyday observation has shown that she can see very well. But at the age of two years and nine months she would not look into the eyes of anyone. She was severely autistic, making no human relationships except to use people as cuddle machines or romping machines, she did not speak and she showed such severe auditory avoidance that she mostly functioned as severely deaf. She has slowly improved over the years, and all these symptoms are now (at the age of five) much improved. She makes a more normal relationship with the nurses and has begun to make relationships with the children. Recently some of the younger nurses have doubted whether she is properly diagnosed as autistic.

This case is a more than usually extreme example of the visual avoidance which is shown to some extent and at some time or other by practically all autistic children. It is probably not without importance that the same symptom is shown by normal children from time to time, and also, indeed, by normal adults.

FAILURE TO RESPOND TO TACTILE OR PAINFUL STIMULI

Autistic children frequently fail to respond to tactile stimuli. When they are in a severely withdrawn state, one can very often touch them in order to attract their attention but evoke no response whatever. Nobody ever accuses these children of having lost the sense of touch or the ability to feel things because at times it is quite obvious they can feel everything normally and they make great use of their tactile sense in manipulating their familiar objects. Indeed many of them get most of their pleasure from the feel of surfaces and textures. An interesting example was that of a boy whose mother had rubella a little less than three months after conception. The child was brought for treatment on account of severe visual and auditory impairment with mental subnormality. There was indeed some visual impairment but the child could see well enough to pick up tiny objects from the carpet at normal range, and it was clear that at times he was disinclined to use all the vision he had. He also functioned as totally deaf when first seen. The examiner produced a tuning fork whilst sitting behind the boy and out of his range of vision. The tuning fork was made to vibrate and was advanced towards the boy's right ear. There was no response. The tuning fork, vibrating strongly, was now advanced towards the left ear. Again there was no response. The tuning fork was again made to vibrate strongly and was advanced towards the right ear; this time however the prongs of the tuning fork were pushed into the child's hair without actually touching his scalp. Still there was no response, although anyone with normal tactile sensibility can feel the vibration of a tuning fork applied to his hair. Even when the tuning fork actually touched his skin he still made no response. Yet the child was at that very moment manipulating objects in such a way as to demand considerable use of sense of touch. There was no suggestion that this child lacked tactile sensibility, but he was accused of being deaf.

If he could feel the tuning fork but did not respond, was there a possibility that he could also hear the tuning fork, yet failed to respond?

A similar phenomenon is the loss of pain sensibility in certain autistic children. These children appear at times to ignore painful stimuli though there is no question of their having true sensory loss to this modality. Recently a child has been brought to the clinic because other children were kicking her and sticking pins in her, producing scars and bruises, without the child's appearing to feel any pain. The mother said that the child never had felt pain and had sat and watched while a skin graft was performed on her own body without anaesthetic. She gave countless other examples, and in the clinic the child ran into the corner of the desk so forcibly as to knock herself over, but then got up and ran on without apparently flinching. This little girl, who was seven years of age, was selectively mute—she would say nothing until the very end of the interview although she talked normally at home—and at times she ignored the spoken word although obviously was not deaf. There was no question of any loss of touch sensation, or indeed of loss of any other sensory modality. An investigation of her peripheral nerves has shown no evidence of neuropathy or neuritis except that the response was not normal in the sensory fibres running in the motor nerve to the orbicularis occuli muscle. Here, then, is a case in which the peripheral nerves are certainly healthy enough to convey pain sensibility, and indeed do so, but in which the child fails to respond to the pain stimuli which must be reaching the brain. This child is not completely withdrawn or autistic, but it seems possible that her failure to respond to painful stimuli may be a species of dissociation or of selective withdrawal from this kind of stimulus. It is of course well known that autistic children and schizophrenic adults are liable to acquire serious burns of the legs through standing too close to radiators, and this danger always has to be borne in mind in mental hospitals.

INTELLECTUAL RETARDATION

An objection commonly made against applying the term schizophrenia to these psychotic or autistic or withdrawn children is that they nearly always function as mentally defective.

It has been suggested that the schizophrenic process will have a much greater disintegrating effect upon the personality if it begins in childhood rather than in adult life, and this might account for many of the clinical differences. A similar effect might be postulated in the intellectual field. It seems doubtful to what extent true dementia occurs in the schizophrenic adult, although the deteriorated case usually has little usefully available intelligence. But the schizophrenic child will nearly always be intellectually retarded, because during the period when his intelligence ought to be developing quickly through the stimulus of new experiences and the interest and inquisitiveness of childhood, the schizophrenic child will lack the desire to interest himself in the real world and how it works and will close his mind against many of the stimuli to which the normal child is especially sensitive (Klein, 1932).

It becomes more and more evident that, in the central nervous system as in other parts of the body, growth and maturation depend very largely upon stimulation (O'Gorman 1968). For normal development, the right stimulus has to be received by the organism at the right time and the right intensity. Visual and auditory avoidance prevent normal access of stimuli to the central nervous system; and 'intellectual avoidance'—the withholding of mental effort—prevents the normal use in intellectual processes of such stimuli as are permitted access. The result must be a relative failure of intellectual growth.

The development of intelligence, it is suggested, depends upon motivation, and upon interest. The withdrawn child is not interested in the world around him and therefore he

89

does not learn about it. He has no incentive to use his intelligence and his intelligence therefore does not develop. Certain things he can and does learn, for example, how to manipulate objects from which he can derive a sensual pleasure, how to open doors and boxes, or to work a gramophone. But if he is not interested in speech or hearing or in any sort of intellectual endeavour then presumably the essential organization of his intellectual faculties does not take place at the appropriate age, or takes place only to a grossly inadequate degree. If, later on, it is possible to persuade the child to enter into the real world and interest himself to some extent in learning and thinking, one would anticipate that it would be too late because he has passed the optimum period of ' learning plasticity ' of his cortex.

Where the withdrawal is only partial, or selective, the patient may be found to have acquired a certain skill, often to a very high degree, whilst the remainder of his intelligence lags far behind. This is the feature referred to as ' partial preservation '. For example, the children may retain their skill in manipulations or their memories may still be good. Some retain their ability to feed daintily and often they can respond to handicraft training although the mental age on testing would be several years below that at which such skills are usually learnt. The commonest example is of course in the field of music and there are many instances of the piano-playing schizophrenic who functions as grossly defective in other fields. Perhaps it was patients of this kind who were in other times referred to as ' idiots savants '; and perhaps, following the same line of thought, we can wonder whether grossly uneven educational or intellectual levels in individuals are as often to be explained by emotional factors resulting in selective withdrawal as by specific organic disabilities.

The suggestion is that an intelligent child may, for emotional reasons like antipathy towards a teacher, decline to interest himself in a particular field of learning, as the result of which his intellectual development in that field may be impaired.

He has in fact *selectively withdrawn* from this field. This phenomenon of selective withdrawal or ' shut off ' is, of course, familiar to all teachers, and occurs, to some extent, in most normal children. Equally important, and much more devasting to the development of the individual's general intelligence, is *partial withdrawal* from reality as a whole, which we see in schizophrenic children.

As suggested above, it seems possible that the phenomena of selective withdrawal, and partial generalized withdrawal, may be of very great importance in the wider academic field. A great many normal people have passed through a period of partial withdrawal during childhood as the result of some emotional upset, but have subsequently recovered. If the withdrawal has persisted at a time when some particular phase of intellectual growth ought to have been proceeding, this may account for some of the blind spots seen in highly intelligent people; and perhaps partial withdrawal during childhood may result in attainment of only mediocre intellectual standards in a person whose initial potential intelligence was very high (O'Gorman, 1954, 1968).

An instructive case from this point of view was that of a soldier referred to the psychiatric centre by his unit medical officer as mentally defective. He could not master the basic essentials of drill, he could not look after his kit, he could not be trusted to do any job assigned to him although he appeared to be willing and to try hard. For this reason he was almost constantly on disciplinary charges. He had no friends and was the butt of his peers. Examination revealed that on testing he had an intelligence quotient in excess of 140. He was a brilliant mathematician, an excellent chess player and was well read in philosophy, upon which he could converse with great knowledge and assurance. However, whilst in the psychiatric centre he continued to be solitary, he made no friends and he was still unable to comply with the very lax disciplinary demands made upon convalescent soldiers.

If the child excludes one field of experience or activity, then neighbouring fields will be affected too. The child who ignores the spoken word, for example, will not himself learn to speak normally, and if he is not using verbal symbols his thinking will be correspondingly handicapped. He will not learn to read or write, so there is a progressive limitation of the fields in which his mind can develop. Moreover, if he does not learn these essential activities at the right time it will not be possible for him to do so properly later on, even if his emotional state improves, because the essential ' cerebral plasticity ' will have been lost. This is one of the reasons why it is often difficult to distinguish subnormality from schizophrenia. A child who shows psychotic mannerisms may be held to be ' defective first with psychosis superimposed ', but perhaps the truth may be that he is ' schizophrenic first, and, as a result, defective '. Even in the case of the child who is said to have always been defective we may wonder whether the child has, in truth, always been schizophrenic. Certainly as our clinical experience enlarges we are seeing younger and younger children who show symptoms which do not differ fundamentally from those shown by rather older children in whom we confidently diagnose schizophrenia (Case No. 1). They have the same inertia, the same lack of interest in those around them and the same lack of warmth. They display, in a similar form, the same sort of mannerisms. They are grossly retarded when first seen and they may remain retarded to a greater or lesser degree. But, just as the older schizophrenic child who improves may suddenly begin to speak in sentences or phrases rather than in single words, so these children may emerge to some extent from their withdrawal and may suddenly begin to walk or play or feed themselves, in a manner more or less appropriate to their chronological age.

MANNERISMS AND ABNORMALITIES OF MOVEMENT

It has been suggested above that these children, having little interest in the world and its people, turn towards their own bodies and their primitive sensory satisfactions for occupation.

All human beings have, unless they are severely ill physically, a continually replenished drive towards activity—an '*elan vitale*'. In the normal child, this is directed into something purposeful like learning or fighting or playing games of imagination. But the autistic child will have none of this. He is not concerned with people and their doings or feelings, so of course he does not play games in which he imagines himself or others doing something in the real world—or in a fantasy world based on reality. Similarly, he does not want to compete with children to whom he is indifferent; or to acquire knowledge about a world in which he is not involved; or to learn skills just because these are of interest to a loved human being—he does not love any human being.

But he must do something. No child can sit motionless all day. He has all this energy, and he has to do something with it. So he occupies himself with any kind of bodily activity or stimulation which gives him pleasure but does not involve participation in reality. From this results most the remaining symptomatology of the condition. Thus, they indulge in rhythmic movements such as rocking, and in bizarre mannerisms. They like to play with water or soil, pouring the material endlessly through their fingers or from one container to another. Often they play with their own excreta and frequent masturbation is very common. ✳ They tend to be preoccupied with surfaces, particularly those which are smooth and cool. They may smell everything or taste everything with which they come into contact, or they may play tricks with the focussing of their own eyes. Often they are fascinated by shadows, or by flickering lights, and we see them shaking their fingers in front of their eyes or looking at objects from odd angles.

Where they are interested in objects these children are interested in the object itself rather than its function in real life, for example they play inappropriately with toys or use implements for purposes other than those for which they are intended. Thus, a propelling pencil might be used simply for the pleasure of screwing or unscrewing it and taking it to pieces. They tend to use people as tools. For example, one may have little or no emotional contact with one of these children yet the child may present himself as soon as he sees the doctor or nurse for a cuddle, using the adult as a sort of cuddling machine for the sensual gratification rather than seeking any true affection. Alternatively, the child may seize the adult's arm and pull him towards the object which he wishes to be manipulated, for example, the door handle or the music box. Their liking for primitive sensations is to be seen in their delight at being swung round or thrown in the air, and many of them have a love of spinning either themselves or the objects with which they play. Usually they love water, and on the whole our children are happiest in the bathing pool. But here again their play tends to be solitary even though they are crowded together.

Compulsive mannerisms, such as sock pulling, nose picking and grunting are also common. Grimacing is almost a routine symptom. Rarely, the grimaces appear to be in response to auditory or visual hallucinations. Mannerisms and attitudes, often of the most bizarre nature, are very common. The head may be rotated a little and sit at an odd angle on the shoulders, which may themselves be unevenly disposed. The hands in repose are held in odd positions, perhaps with the fingers at different angles, and the wrists unduly flexed. The child may sit for long periods with the trunk bent forward or sideways in seemingly uncomfortable postures, with the legs similarly disposed. More often than not, movements are as well co-ordinated as those of normal children, but some of the deteriorated patients walk with an odd, shambling gait or bend down and up again with each stride, or hold their arms stiffly away from their sides with elbows flexed, and feet turned widely out. In some cases the child's abnormal posture or gait, if sustained for months or years, may cause anatomical changes in and around the affected joints leading, for example, to kyphosis or to deformities around the knees and ankles.

There are countless other peculiarities of movement, no two children being exactly alike. ' Sudden run ' describes the mannerism of suddenly breaking into an aimless gallop for a few yards and then standing motionless. This is of course a typical example of a mannerism which may be exhibited by schizophrenics of all ages. Rocking is perhaps the commonest mannerism of all, and head banging is often seen. In the most deteriorated cases ' head bashing ', with one or both hands, or self mutilation by biting or picking may occur. This is the most distressing symptom for those who look after the children, and perhaps the hardest to explain. Possibly it may be a desperate means of excluding reality, for it occurs most often when the child is thwarted in any way, or particularly anxious. A normal man, emotionally in extremis, may dig his nails into his palms—presumably to provide a strong stimulus to distract him from the agony he is enduring. Perhaps these children are trying to exclude unpleasant reality by filling their sensorium with a painful stimulus which they have learned to tolerate and which they can, at least, control. This of course is an hypothesis which will be very difficult to prove. But if one watches one of these children for long periods trying to beat or mutilate himself, it is hard indeed to convince oneself that the symptom arises from an ' unawareness of his own personal identity '.

Another common reaction to frustration is toneless and prolonged screaming or roaring. Having no interest in people they do not have social consciences to tell them they have cried or screamed for long enough. In the same way, expressions of pleasure tend to be exaggerated through lack of inhibition. These children tense their bodies and shake with delight in a mannerism described as ' squeezy shudder ' but which is an exaggeration of a mannerism seen in many normal children.

Pulling the lips up into a snout, narrowing the eyes, or

looking upwards and sideways are among facial mannerisms seen, and diagnostically the most important is 'looking through' a person—gazing at him with apparently unseeing eyes with no evident flicker of emotion.

PSYCHOSOMATIC SYMPTOMS

Autistic children are prone to a variety of physical symptoms, with some there is controversy as to whether emotional disturbances are responsible for physical up-sets or vice versa; perhaps both positions are valid.

Case No. 13. Matthew. Admitted to Smiths Hospital, aged 6 years.

Early History—Seven weeks premature (birthweight 4 lb. 8 oz.). Forceps delivery; anoxia at birth, pneumonia and septicaemia as neonate; nursed in oxygen intermittently; born with a poorly developed lower jaw; unable to swallow; tube fed from birth until admission to Smiths; tube was passed by nurses and then by his mother three times a day. At Great Ormond Street Hospital, aged 3 months, he was considered to be suffering from facial and palatal paresis and inability to swallow; a flaccid baby who suffered from apnoea and had to be nursed in oxygen; subsequently admitted to hospital for dysphagia, ' deafness ', iron deficiency anaemia, bronchitis and pneumonia; jaw remained grossly under-developed but teething normal.

On Admission—Severely psychotic, withdrawn, negativistic, manneristic, speechless (but made complicated noises). Though he had been thought to be deaf it was now evident that he could hear normally. His failure to swallow was not complete—both his parents has seen him swallow occasionally; moreover, he not only failed to swallow—he refused to take anything into his mouth except the tube for his feeds. The only exception to this was an occasional sip of water which he would swallow in hot weather. But usually, when he let a little water trickle into his mouth, he coughed it all back again as soon as it reached the posterior one-third of his tongue. Following extensive and expert investigation when he was 7 years old it was reported; ' Apart from his unwillingness to swallow and a complete pharyngeal palsy, his swallowing mechanism seems to be intact. If he were willing to swallow there seems to be no reason why he should not take food by mouth provided this is not of a dry nature and is washed down with liquid. . . . However, I do think he has a genuine pharyngeal palsy. His inability to swallow when you put material into his pharynx is a voluntary act but when he does make his swallowing motion then I do not think he could possibly inhibit his pharyngeal constrictors while compensating for the defect with his tongue. His larynx closes and his cricopharyngeus opens at the right stage. It is not uncommon to find partial or complete pharyngeal palsies in children who swallow normally and in whom they have never been suspected. I have not seen this type of thing in anyone who might be regarded as psycho-neurotic or " hysterical " '.

Matthew even failed to swallow his saliva, so that even though his bib was changed frequently and his clothing he (and anyone who came near him) was continually smeared extensively with evil-smelling mucus so that it was difficult for anyone to cuddle him. Yet he loved being cuddled, even though he did not make a relationship with the adult whom he seemed to regard simply as a ' cuddle-machine '. He showed manual dexterity, when so minded, which indicated that he had more intelligence than he used; but he was functioning at idiot level. Slowly the feeding tube was withdrawn; but such was his resistance to swallowing food that he tended to become emaciated and the tube had to be used again. Eventually he was induced to take a normal diet and to swallow most of his saliva, though he continued to dribble occasionally. At 8 years he developed a limp which was inconstant, disappearing when he hurried, and he could do other things, like jumping on a trampoline or climbing in the gymnasium, without apparent difficulty. The orthopaedic surgeon regarded the limp as ' functional ' but it persisted; eventually the leg was put in plaster; when this was taken off after several weeks the limp was much improved, though it tended to recur when he was unwilling to walk. His neck was remarkably thin, and he preferred to rest his head on the table or support it with his hand in his neck. He was given a rigid collar which did not support his head but prevented him from supporting it with his hand, and the strength of his neck and the length of time during which he would hold up his head improved.

At $3\frac{1}{2}$ years Matthew eats well but often retains food; this he works up into a bolus which he seems able to swallow and then regurgitate into his mouth. He limps slightly but he can run, climb, skate and kick a football—his one real contact with other human beings occurs when he plays football. Manual dexterity is good. He handles a pencil and scissors well and can draw lines with a ruler or stencil; but apart from that he only scribbles. He can match pictures and do fairly complicated jig-saw puzzles but it is difficult to get him to do anything. He prefers to sit by the radiator, his head in the crook of his arm. In the swimming pool he appeared to be about to learn to swim but was excluded because of faecal incontinence, which he does not show at other times. There is no speech and no pre-speech sounds. He shows visual and auditory avoidance and 'motor avoidance' when one attempts to direct his hand.

Polydipsia (excessive drinking) is common. One child, if prevented from drinking, became very distressed and his intake and output of fluid was enormous. It was suggested that 'pitressin-insensitive diabetes insipidus' was the diagnosis, since posterior-pituitary preparations did not help. Lately there has been some improvement in his autistic symptoms and in his excessive drinking. Perhaps the polydipsia was initially an autistic mannerism. But it is easy to imagine, by analogy with what is known to happen with other endocrine glands, that the function of the posterior pituitary, as regulator of water balance, might have been altered by the abnormal stimulation offered to the gland by the excessive drinking—eventually he might come to need excessive quantities of fluid because of functional changes in the gland.

Disturbances of growth and metabolism in autistic children have been described in Chapter 4 (*pp. 55 et seq*). At this point it is of interest to consider further the interaction of emotional and physical disturbances. If psycho-somatic illness in non-psychotic patients is any guide, one would not be surprised to find that circular mechanisms are involved, emotional disability aggravating physical dysfunction which in turn causes a worsening of the emotional state. There are many observations which indicate that growth depends upon stimulation, as already emphasised (p. 89). Suppose an autistic child received insufficient maternal stimulation initially, and that he later cut down the amount of stimulation he accepted (through withdrawal or dissociation) then the stimulation necessary, not only for intellectual growth but also for physical development might be deficient; and this might have something to do with the physical immaturity of many of our patients. All of this is, of course, no more than speculation. But experiments to test such hypotheses might not be too difficult to carry out.

Squint is also common. Usually it is inconstant, varying with the presence or absence of certain people or the degree of disturbance at the time, and alternating between one eye and the other. Nearly always it is internal. Squint is considered an indication that the child's condition is due to 'organic' disease. The opposite point of view seems worth considering, namely that emotional disturbance may be the cause of squint.

CHAPTER 6

THE NATURE OF AUTISM

There is no reason to suppose that the phenomenon of dissociation operates only in respect of auditory or visual stimuli. Evidence quoted above suggests that sensory stimuli of other modalities—touch, pain, temperature, smell—are similarly cut off or dissociated. There is no doubt that any kind of sensory stimulus can be dissociated, for this is one of the key mechanisms of the hysteric and one is used to seeing adults who are hysterically blind, hysterically deaf, hysterically insensitive to pain or even to touch. Presumably this is what happens under hypnotic suggestion, when for therapeutic or dramatic purposes various sensory stimuli, especially pain, can be effectively excluded in the conscious but susceptible subject.

Yet it must not be imagined that the mechanism of dissociation is in itself necessarily pathological. On the contrary, it is probably one of the most essential of all cerebral mechanisms, for it is necessary that the human being should be able to dissociate various sensory stimuli; otherwise, these would obtrude and prevent the individual from concentrating on the matter in hand. If one is attempting to compose or converse or read and one needs to concentrate, one has to be able to exclude extraneous stimuli. Without this power of dissociation nobody would be able to work in the pandemonium that occurs in many large offices. Most of us, in fact, dissociate (or are withdrawn from) 90 per cent of our sensory environment for 90 per cent of the time.

The faculty for dissociation can, of course, be specific; that is to say, stimuli from one particular source may be allowed free access whilst other stimuli of the same modality are excluded. Perhaps this is the mechanism by which mother can be in a very deep sleep, oblivious to the sounds of thunderstorms, or conjugal snores or nearby revelry, but awaken immediately the baby begins to cry. This power of selective dissociation is perhaps the mechanism behind the selective withdrawal seen so often in autistic children. They will respond to some sounds, and not to others, or to some peoples' voices and not others.

The power of dissociation, it would appear, is not limited merely to incoming sensory stimuli. We must also be able to shut off various distracting thoughts or memories or even instinctual needs if we are trying to concentrate upon a particular subject. Indeed, if it were not possible at any one time to exclude from consciousness all but a very small range of our memories, fears, hopes and preoccupations, then useful and constructive thought would be impossible. The mechanism of dissociation cannot, therefore, be confined specifically to the neural connections between the hypothalamus and the frontal cortex. It must be available at many other sites in the brain, and perhaps universally in that organ.

What is being suggested, in fact, is that dissociation, or withdrawal, is not merely a normal, but a basic and essential function of the mind; and that in this function of dissociation we have the mechanism not merely of the deafness and failure to respond to pain stimuli of the autistic child, but also of the withdrawal which is the essential characteristic of his condition. He can withdraw from or dissociate sounds, sights, smells, pains, touches and memories, just as he can withdraw from people. He can also withdraw from various faculties such as speaking, reading, learning, or even thinking constructively. He can be withdrawn from one, or two, or several of these senses or functions or thoughts, completely or partially. (This is selective, or partially selective, withdrawal or dissociation.) He can be completely withdrawn from a very large number of functions (in which case we would describe him as completely withdrawn or completely autistic), or he can be partially withdrawn from the whole of reality (in which case he could be also described as incompletely autistic or, perhaps, moderately schizophrenic).

What has to be emphasized is that it is not only recognizably autistic children who withdraw. Everybody withdraws, because everybody has to; and the phenomenon cannot therefore be described as being of itself abnormal. A normal child in a brown study is withdrawn; a person immersed in a book, who fails to respond to a remark or a conversation in the same room, is withdrawn for the time being from that kind of auditory stimulus; but if the dinner gong sounds, he may hear it. The suggestion is that what has happened in cases like that of Freddie (Case No. 12) is that they withdrew from a range of auditory stimuli in infancy and, because of their emotional states, continued to do so until this became a habit. Having no effective hearing during the time when they were supposed to be learning to talk, they could not, of course, acquire this skill; and they might, in any case, withdraw also from the whole activity of communication, so that their speechlessness might be both directly and indirectly attributed to selective withdrawal. Perhaps, in Ellen's case (Case No. 11), there was withdrawal not only from hearing and communication, but also from other fields of experience and activity; and perhaps when the environment became too threatening or obtrusive she made an almost complete withdrawal—into a truly autistic state—for the time being.

It could be said that the ability to withdraw is an inborn propensity, highly developed in early infancy; that the facility for developing this propensity is greatest in the highly pliable days of early childhood; and that, just as a blind child trained intensively to use his sense of touch from his earliest days, will continue to make the greatest possible use of that faculty as part of his way of life, so the unstimulated or threatened infant who from his earliest days makes maximum use of the faculty to withdraw is likely to continue to do so, and in effect, to make excessive withdrawal an essential part of his way of life. Or the situation could be described from a different point of view by saying that infants have to be tempted into involvement with people and with their world by appropriate stimulation and by various instinctual satisfactions. If they are not so stimulated and rewarded, or if, on the contrary, they feel themselves threatened by the environment, then the propensity for normal involvement with reality will not be developed.

This, then, is the fourth of the methods of coping with unacceptable reality described briefly in Chapter 3. The mechanism of withdrawal (selective withdrawal) is what is employed in the hysteric. The affectionless psycopath also uses (partial) withdrawal as his mechanism of defence. In fact, in the present writer's view, the excessive use of the second, third and fourth normal methods of defence against unacceptable reality—i.e. adoption of obsessions and rituals, distortion of reality and withdrawal from reality—constitute a very large part indeed of what we regard as mental illness.

CHAPTER 7

THE PSEUDO-SCHIZOPHRENIC SYNDROMES

The suggestion that the essence of autism is withdrawal or non-involvement, and that autism is best regarded as a symptom rather than a disease or even a syndrome, may perhaps be of use in reaching some understanding of some syndromes which might otherwise have been regarded as clinical conditions, *sui generis*, just as Heller's syndrome and Mahler's syndrome and so many other conditions which show autism as their main feature have been described as distinct clinical entities. In general, of course, it is probably true that every child is a special syndrome of his own; nevertheless, it is convenient to group certain cases together by virtue of some outstanding points of clinical similarity.

THE ACUTELY DEPRIVED CHILD

Reference has already been made to the kind of patient, so accurately described by Bowlby (1951) in which the child, separated suddenly from his mother by some catastrophe such as admission to hospital or death of the parent, becomes inert, listless, and disinterested in his surroundings or in his attendants. This work, which has been the foundation of recent efforts to secure frequent visiting of children in hospitals, has been supported by important observations on animals, particularly on monkeys, which has shown that when deprived of their mothers, or even of their familiar toys, and then placed in unfamiliar surroundings, baby monkeys will lie down inertly and refuse to play or to interest themselves at all in their environment.

Usually the children suffering from this acute deprivation syndrome have been described as depressed, and indeed this is an accurate description of their mood. There is, however, a strong element of withdrawal in such children and in these cases the withdrawal might be described as a symptom of the depression. There is nothing essentially different, in their withdrawal, from the withdrawal shown by children diagnosed autistic or schizophrenic, except that the condition nearly always arises from a fairly rapid and definite deprivation, and that the prognosis is in most cases very good provided that the familiar attendant and familiar surroundings are quickly restored, or that an adequate substitute mother and a supporting new environment can be provided. Speaking in the language used in the previous chapter, we would say that these children are generally and severely withdrawn, but as a rule only temporarily. In some cases, however, prolonged or repeated deprivations of this kind seem to result in the formation of a habit of withdrawal when confronted with adverse circumstances; and some degree of withdrawal may become a way of life in these children. Of course the condition is not confined to children; it is common knowledge that a severely depressed adult may take little or no interest in his surroundings, being physically and mentally inert and often complaining that he is unable to make a relationship with anybody. As he gets better he begins to take an interest. In the adult, of course, the withdrawal is rarely complete, but every psychiatrist who has had the extremely difficult task of distinguishing between a catatonic stupor in an adult schizophrenic, and a depressive stupor in a patient with severe melancholia knows that in the main he must be guided by the history and the subsequent behaviour of the patient in making his diagnosis.

Perhaps the tendency of the symptom of withdrawal to occur in various kinds of emotional illness may account for some of the difficulties in diagnosis both in adult and in children's psychiatry.

PSEUDO-SCHIZOPHRENIA OF TWINS

The exceedingly close relationship of many twins, particularly identical twins, is well known. Often the parents of twins express some concern because the children take very little interest in anyone except each other. This situation is very grossly exaggerated in some cases in which two apparently severely psychotic twins showing some or all of the diagnostic criteria suggested in the ' Nine Points ' described in Chapter 1 are brought to the clinic for advice or treatment. Nearly always these children are backward, especially in speech. On close observation, however, it becomes evident that the children do communicate, but only with each other. Their communication does not rely on ordinary words, but on grunts and gestures and laughter and screams and action. They seem to have a kind of communication very reminiscent of intelligent young monkeys. Some of the mothers of these children acquire considerable insight into this bizarre communication, and the twins may communicate with her in the same way. It transpires that the twins are interested only in each other and in their mother; and their interest in mother seems to be rather less than is usual. These children tend to be very over-active and unbiddable and they make little or no relationship with other children. All their emotional interest, hate as well as love, rivalry as well as support, seems to be concentrated on each other. A typical case is described below.

Case No. 14. Beryl and Gillian. Admitted to Smiths Hospital aged four years and nine months

History—They are monozygotic twins. The pregnancy was normal except that mother was said to have some ' heart trouble '. The labour and birth were normal. Gillian weighed 6 lb. 12 oz., Beryl 5 lb. 8 oz. They were breast fed for only a few days because the doctor did not think mother's health good enough for her to continue to feed them. In fact, they were the seventh and eighth children of a family who at that time were all under 14 years. Material circumstances in the family were not good and their mother, who was under the care of the doctor because of physical and 'nervous' symptoms, had great difficulty in coping with her large family.

The twins were said to have sat up ' fairly early ' but the health visitor noted they were not walking at 15 months. At 19 months they were crawling and by two years both were walking, although at that time Gillian was a little behind Beryl. At the age of two and a half they were brought to the paediatrician because one had symptoms suggesting scurvy and the other of rickets. They were in a wretched condition which was described by the paediatrician when they were three years ten months as follows. ' These children are very withdrawn even from each other and have many mannerisms, frantic temper outbursts and a number of traits commonly seen in psychotic children.' A few months later he thought that there had been some improvement; they could ' hardly be said to be withdrawn from each other but they are still withdrawn from adults '. Their mother said that they screamed incessantly, that their behaviour was wild and unmanageable, that they were a very great trial in the home, and that she was quite exhausted.

Beryl was admitted to a general hospital at the age of four and a half where she was diagnosed as suffering from acute pyelonephritis with meningism and as being a psychotic child. She was said to whimper continuously and occasionally emit piercing screams. ' Behaves like a caged animal; completely withdrawn from all human contact; repetitive actions for up to two hours. Behaviour impossible.'

On admission to Smiths Hospital both were considered to be undernourished. Gillian was considered to be brighter than her twin. Both spoke but were said to be doubly incontinent. Beryl tended to bully Gillian and was the more disturbed of the two, given to long periods of screaming and crying and temper tantrums. They spoke very little but screamed almost continuously, refusing all efforts by staff to make a relationship with them. A few days after admission they were noted as having ' cheered up enormously '. They still smelt everything and rubbed things against their upper lips and ignored the spoken word. Their speech was at the level of a child of about two years, consisting of monosyllables and also occasional phrases like ' dickey bird gone '. There followed a phase during which there was increased withdrawal, the twins taking little notice even of one another. This lasted only a few weeks, however, and they began to make relationships with the staff and were more friendly towards one another.

A few weeks after this they began to make relationships with other children and their play became progressively more normal.

Within three months they had acquired sphincter control, had only occasional bouts of screaming, and were generally less unruly. They were showing much more decipherable speech, whereas previously they had seemed to communicate only with each other. Now, also, they were beginning to have relationships with other children as well as with members of the staff, whereas previously they had taken no notice of anyone except to scream when approached; even their aggressiveness had been directed only against each other. They were improving physically. The reports of the nursing staff show that they were no longer functioning as low grade mentally subnormal children. They went to the hospital school and began to show some signs of responding to education. A year after admission they began to attend the local infants' school and continued to do so for one year, following which, at the age of eight years, they were discharged to their own home. However, they had to be re-admitted to Smiths four months later because neither the home nor the school could cope with them. Very soon, however, they were back at the junior school in town which they continued to attend until they were ten years old. It is of interest that their intellectual level on testing fell a little after the unsuccessful attempt at living at home (*see* Table 3).

TABLE 3

Psychological Assessments

Terman Merrill			Weschler Intelligence Scale for Children—Performance		
Chronological age	Intelligence quotient		Chronological age	Intelligence quotient	
	Beryl	Gillian		Beryl	Gillian
4 : 9	47	49	5 : 10	93	108
5 : 9	51	68	7 : 0	89	86
5 : 10	60	74	7 : 10	106	90
7 : 0	73	80	9 : 0	85	89
7 : 10	77	81	10 : 1	91	90
9 : 0	72	76			
10 : 1	75	81			

An electroencephalograph carried out when they were nine years and three months showed an identical record for both twins. This was described as being ' outside normal limits and showing features of almost epileptoid type on over-breathing '. There was no significant change on an EEG carried out five months later.

Physically, both twins showed steady improvement throughout their period under the hospital's care and subsequently. The only physical abnormality of note was that both children were found to have nystagmus which later disappeared.

After leaving Smiths Hospital, aged ten years and three months, they spent one year at a special residential school and were then transferred to another. They made steady, normal progress and at about their 13th birthday they were found to be two rather hilarious and slightly backward teenagers whose behaviour was rather uninhibited and whose relationships with both adults and other youngsters was warm and immediate, though perhaps on a somewhat superficial plane; but they would certainly both have been described within normal limits emotionally.

Such children as these might be described as being sufficient unto each other. There is from the beginning a triangular relationship between them and their mother and, particularly in a large family or with a mother who does not take special pains to treat the children very much as individuals, the two may be left very much to their own mutual devices, so that a very close relationship evolves which is in fact pathological. Having each other, they do not need other people. If they do not form relationships with other people, then, it is suggested, they are likely to lack the urge to concern themselves with the real world of other people. It would not be true in these cases to say that each child lives in a world of his own; they live in a world of each other. Consequently they can have little desire to advance in the real world, little need for the approval of their mother for any forward step they may take, much less the approval of anyone else. They do not need to talk because they can make their requirements known to each other, and to a lesser extent to their mother, and they do not want anything from other people. They make up their own games without reference to the games of other children, and they have little need to compete with them.

Beryl and Gillian showed a most remarkable improvement under treatment aimed at persuading them to regard themselves as separate individuals rather than identical halves of the same person. Under normal conditions, and even without treatment, such twins would eventually become separated somehow or other and the prognosis tends to be very much better than in the case of most autistic children.

George and Thomas (Case No. 15) provide an exception to this generalization. They are identical twins who apparently developed normally at first and were walking unaided at 14 months. After this, however, their development appeared to slow down, and, though they began to say single words at about 18 months and acquired the expected number of words by about 2 years, they never used phrases and learned no more words after about $2\frac{1}{2}$ years. Moreover, at this time, mother noticed they were not looking at her as her other children had done and were less responsive to sounds, whereas for the first 2 years they had appeared much more sensitive to noise than their siblings. By the age of 4 years they had become overactive and showed visual and auditory avoidance, inconstant squint and a growing number of mannerisms. They no longer spoke except for odd words, they never acquired control of bowels or bladder, they made no relationships with other children. They did take notice of one another, although not sufficiently to be able to play any sort of game, and they enjoyed cuddles and romps with mother and with the siblings—all of whom were girls, older than themselves, and devoted to the twins. It was of interest that mother considered father had been inordinately jealous of the twins from their birth and he was quite unable to tolerate their behaviour. However, mother insisted on keeping them at home and they were contained during the daytime at the local training centre. At the age of 9 years they are grossly hyperactive, mischievous, unbiddable, wordless, and impossible to occupy constructively. The prognosis in this case must be poor indeed.

PSEUDO-SCHIZOPHRENIC NEGATIVISM

A group of cases which show a remarkable resemblance to cases of the schizophrenic syndrome, and from which they are not usually distinguished, are those in which there exists extreme negativism towards the parents, in particular the mother, throughout childhood. These are children who do not associate with their contemporaries, who function as subnormal although from time to time they show glimpses of intelligence at a much higher level, and who are grossly dependent and babyish. The key to this condition lies perhaps in the fact that they are always very much worse when their mothers are present; they seem to punish and torment their mothers through their stupidity and extreme cloying dependence. If they are separated from their mothers they indulge in most violent tantrums before and at the moment of separation, but their violent distress abates rapidly after mother has departed.

The situation usually occurs in girls rather than boys, and it seems as though the child is trying to use her babyishness as a means of concentrating all the interest and attention of both parents exclusively upon herself. The fathers always show a great affection towards the child and a total inability to treat her with any firmness. The mothers show an extraordinary mixture of affection and resentment; they tolerate the most extreme provocation from the child, cleaning up after her, putting up with her violent tantrums, allowing her to make normal family life impossible. They try, usually with a good deal of success, to mask both from themselves and from the rest of the world their resentment of the child's behaviour. The parents go frantically from paediatrician to psychiatrist, from medical to non-medical hypnotist, from faith healer to quack, in an effort to find someone who will produce a ' cure ' for their daughter. Nobody can help them very much because the only treatment which has any chance of success is early removal from the family, and a gradual reintroduction, depending entirely on how well the child is prepared to behave when at home. And the parents, all of whom suffer from a severe degree of what Ounsted has called ' hyper-pedophilia ' are unable to accept this drastic treatment. The more distressing the symptoms are to the mother the more will the child persist in them.

Sometimes the children show functional deafness or mutism as described in the schizophrenic syndrome, and this too they seem to use as a weapon, valuable because it distresses the parents and relieves the child from the responsibility of learning or growing up. Usually the child cannot be separated from the mother because of the extreme emotional involvement she has with the child and the patients become mentally defective adolescents and adults, as dependent on their mothers as sick babies. Their relationship is very like the symbiotic relationship described by Mahler, persisting through infancy into childhood and adult life. Perhaps, however, it should be described as a parasitic rather than a symbiotic relationship, because it is destructive to the mother and therefore, ultimately, to the child.

These children show most of the symptoms described as criteria of the schizophrenic syndrome by the Working Party (Creak, 1961)—failure to form personal relationships, functional subnormality, difficulties in communication and hearing, odd mannerisms and psychosomatic dysfunction. Yet one is left with the very strong impression that the illness is one of the family as a whole rather than of the single patient. The children do not have quite the same emotional ' feel ' as the truly autistic child. One can make a relationship with them—or one could, were it not that they refuse to be drawn away from the parents. One can, once they are removed from the parents, persuade them to give up many of their psychotic

112

symptoms. Sometimes, in fact, they do well in hospital, provided the parents leave them alone. But usually the parents cannot do this, and thus the child continues his habitual imitation of the irresponsible baby even in hospital, and the pattern may be prolonged as an indelible habit of behaviour. A typical case is described below.

Case No. 16. June. Admitted to Smiths Hospital at the age of seven years and ten months

Mother's complaint—Unmanageable at home and on the way to school; backwardness; tantrums; failure to make friends.

History—The parents claimed that pregnancy, labour and early history were in all respects normal, in fact, June was somewhat precocious and passed all her milestones early. At three years of age she started nursery school across the close from her home in a modern flat. She went and came daily alone, watched by her mother. She settled at once and made friends whom she brought home, and was a generally happy, confident child. When June was four and a half the family moved in order to give her a garden. They kept her at the same nursery school as she seemed so well settled there, although this meant a daily journey both ways by bus. At this stage, however, when mother arrived to fetch her in the afternoons June flew into violent tantrums, screaming and kicking in the bus and in the street all the way home. However, she settled down as soon as she arrived home. At this time also she began to object to being dressed at home to go out anywhere, including school. The misbehaviour on the way home from school eased when mother allowed June to walk on alone. The journey took a full half hour and mother followed unseen. June talked to people and animals whom she met on the way, but arrived home happy and relaxed. However, mother found this a great strain and the next term June was moved to a new nursery school nearer home. Here she never settled well, saying she did not like the teachers or children. She made no friends and became solitary. The school complained that she would not try to learn at all. She still preferred walking home alone, and when her mother fetched her she again showed tantrums all the way home. At times she insisted on being carried, saying her legs ached. Mother became very exhausted. Because of her disturbed behaviour she did not

113

move to the primary school at the age of five, but remained at the nursery. June's behaviour became more and more uncontrolled. In buses she tried to push people off the seats, and in queues she pushed people out of the way. Finally, at the age of about six and a half her parents gave up taking her to school and she remained at home. She resisted being dressed to go out of the house and said she was afraid to do so. The School Attendance Officer's calls were of no avail and June was referred to the Child Guidance Clinic. She was admitted to Smiths Hospital at the age of seven years ten months.

Family history—Mother. The maternal grandmother died when mother was nine years old, and mother was brought up by her own grandmother. She completely lost contact with her father and siblings and left her grandmother at the age of 17 to fend for herself. She is intelligent, fastidious, meticulous, house-proud, ambitious for her daughter and very anxious that the family shall be successful and respected in the community. She seemed to be affectionate and warm towards her daughter but was chronically anxious. *Father.* He suffered much hardship in early life and had a rough, tough upbringing. He is a highly skilled factory worker and is keen on motor-cycles and cars, engineering and all forms of sport. He too is chronically anxious, the anxiety being shown not only in his excessive concern for his daughter but also in various psychosomatic symptoms, mostly gastric and dermatological.

June is an only child and the reason given for this by the parents was that they wished to use all their resources to give June the best possible upbringing. Both parents doted on the child, but they had different ambitions for her. Mother desired a very feminine and fastidious daughter, interested and successful in womanly pursuits, whereas father wanted a tomboy, good at sport and lessons, a child who would be both son and daughter to him and who would achieve, through education and application, the academic, athletic and business success which he himself had desired.

Father was, in fact, pathologically preoccupied with his daughter, and inclined to indulge her in every way, whereas mother wanted to be firm with her and was less sentimentally affectionate towards her. The result was a continuous conflict between the parents which June took every opportunity to exploit. Thus, she developed

114

a skill at setting one person against the other which the Matron has described as 'almost an island of intelligence'. She refused to co-operate with her mother or to make any effort to learn or progress socially at school, or to give up her dependent babyish status. She plagued her mother with continuous repetitious questions and impossible demands, and sought exclusively to occupy her father's time and attention at mother's expense; nor would she permit any show of affection between the parents. At one stage she was insisting that father should sleep in her bed whilst she went in with mother.

From the time of her admission to Smiths Hospital very close contact was maintained with the parents, the Psychiatric Social Worker visiting mother very frequently, and the father regularly seeing the doctor at the psychiatric clinic. It was, however, exceedingly difficult to get father to modify his attitude. Mother attempted to be firm but she was defeated by June's determination and father's weakness and his need for close contact with the child. At first the parents were asked not to visit the hospital so as to give all three a rest from the triangular situation. June made but slow progress at the hospital, refusing to make any effort to learn in school or to make social progress in the group. She continually accused other children of picking on her and made hypochondriacal excuses when asked to do anything.

In hospital she slowly became more amenable and at the age of eight and a half, about eight months after admission, she was described as 'a different child'. She had made good all-round progress and there was a much better relationship between herself and the other children. The parents did not visit during the first few months and when they began visiting again all three members of the family became exceedingly upset on each occasion, so much so that mother ceased visiting and father came alone. In fact, these visits from the parents seemed to be harmful to June's progress. Between visits, she usually behaved calmly and got on fairly well with the other children. She was greedy for individual attention, however, and sought to exclude the other children. Four months later the Matron noted that she was sweet and well behaved in the hospital but a little fiend with her parents. She was always very neat and tidy in her appearance and, although she would make no effort to learn to read or write or do sums at school her handiwork was always described by the teacher as very good. When she was nearly nine an attempt was made to begin to re-introduce her into her own family. Mother could not tolerate visiting the hospital so June was taken home for brief visits, seeing mother and father alternately once a fortnight. However, her progress in the hospital was now practically nil. When she was nine and three-quarters she was noted as being very noisy, as having a variable squint, and as rolling her eyes and rocking. The teacher thought that she was ' losing the true relationship between fantasy and reality, not only through sound but through vision also '. She was always blaming other children if one as much as glanced in her direction. She was again asking repetitive questions. In ten minutes she asked the question ' Is my mummy coming today? ' 25 times although teacher answered ' Yes ' on each occasion. She imagined other children were teasing and hurting her and accused them of hitting her although they might be at the other end of the room. When she was ten she had a sudden improvement in school work though this was mostly confined to handicraft and self-care. Soon afterwards, however, she had a major set-back in her school work and whereas she had learned to write sentences before, now she would not write at all. Her attitude became even more paranoid and she even accused the school books of teasing her.

In spite of her failure to make progress in the hospital, the parents claimed that she was doing much more at home and the policy of slowly returning her to her family was maintained, the visits being increasingly prolonged. Finally, when June was 12 years 10 months old her parents kept her at home, saying they could no longer face the terrible scene which happened whenever they tried to get her to come back to the hospital.

The Psychiatric Social Worker kept in close touch with the family and an attempt was made to introduce her to the local training centre. However, there was no place for her immediately and she remained at home for eight months without occupation or training outside the home. When she got a place at the training centre (aged 14) she made great difficulties about walking up the road to the school bus and kicked and screamed all the way. Her mother persevered and she improved in this respect. At the training centre the staff thought that she was beginning to show some improvement. However, there was a ten day half term holiday and thereafter June refused to return. Neither the parents nor the Mental Welfare Officer could succeed in getting her to return to the centre.

By the time June was 15 years 10 months old an extraordinary situation had developed at home. June dominated the household and constantly ordered her mother about. She would not allow her mother into the living room or kitchen and in fact she took over the ground floor of the house, confining her mother to the upstairs rooms and the garden. She was whining, difficult and obstinate and quite unamenable to any kind of discipline. Nevertheless, she was doing the cooking and cleaning, washing and ironing with remarkable competence, the house being faultlessly clean and father expressing himself as delighted with his food and very proud of his daughter. After father had had his evening meal June would dress herself carefully and persuade him to take her to the cinema or bowling alley or for drives in the car, mother, of course, being left behind. Eventually, mother refused to tolerate the situation any longer and insisted that June be admitted to hospital.

In hospital June's behaviour deteriorated severely and when she was 16 and a half years of age she was described as being unable to dress herself properly, as noisy, boisterous and acting like a severely subnormal child. Her habits were dirty and her manners infantile. When her parents visited her, her behaviour was worse than ever, and the pain which she was causing them was very apparent. However, a new regime was begun in the hospital in which firmer discipline was applied to her than ever before, coupled with a great deal of individual attention and affection. The family had at long last learned that they had to deal firmly with her and by so doing they were able to visit her in hospital and get her to return to the ward after each visit. However, if she was allowed to go home it was only with the most extreme difficulty that she could be got back to the hospital. She has made some progress and her handiwork is now almost as good as it was when she was nine years old. She can wash and dress herself after a fashion, is rather less boisterous except when her parents are present, and will do more or less as she is told.

Her intelligence test results have been remarkably constant all through, within a few points of I.Q. 50 no matter what test was applied or at what age. Her handicraft and housecraft when she was in a good mood and a stable phase were vastly above this level. Physically she has maintained excellent health throughout. Her highly variable squint, which is at times entirely absent, has been the only abnormal physical sign.

Another patient in whom the symptoms of autism are presen. in severe degree but in whom negativism appears to be the most important factor is John (Case No. 17) aged 3 years 11 montht on admission. Problem—does not stand or walk unless mother is holding his hand; severe head-banging and general negativisms

Family history—father is a local government officer, and mother a housewife who does not go out to work. There are two other children, girl aged 10 years and boy aged 6 years, both of them entirely normal. There is no history in the family of formal psychiatric illness.

Personal history—pregnancy, birth and delivery were normal and John was born at home. His birth weight was 9 lbs. He was not breast-fed but accepted the bottle readily. He sat alone at the age of 2 years and learned to stand, when supported, about six months later. He was walking with support by the age of 3 years. At the age of 14 months he was seen by a paediatrician; at that time he was unable to sit unaided and made no attempts to feed himself, did not play with toys and had no speech. He appeared to be hypotonic. He was admitted to hospital and fully investigated but no abnormality was found to account for his retardation. He was then referred to Great Ormond Street Hospital and they, too, found that he was a simple, mentally defective child and were unable to make any suggestions as to treatment.

As an infant John had been excessively quiet, lying in his pram silently for hours, and crying very little. But according to his mother his behaviour deteriorated once he learned to talk and sit up (which he did when he was about 3 years old). He learned to stand and to walk with support early in his fourth year, but would make no attempt to walk unaided. In fact he would only walk when actually touching his mother. His head-banging became much worse and now occurred whenever he was frustrated in any way and there was much bruising of his face and head. Temper tantrums were steadily increasing. Although previously he had often been content to sit quietly with mother and watch television, now he refused to do this. He was becoming increasingly defiant and negativistic—for example, if mother said ' Don't pull the curtains ', this is exactly what John tried to do. The only way mother could get any peace was to put him in his cot with a cover to prevent him from banging his head, and by the time of admission John was spending a considerable proportion of his time in this way. He had begun to say a few words at the age of 3 years and at the time of admission he was talking fairly fluently and using sentences appropriately. There had been no prolonged separations from home except for two admissions to hospital for about a fortnight. At the age of 3 years and 9 months he was seen by a Consultant Psychiatrist who considered that he was both mentally retarded and psychotic and that special treatment was unlikely to prove of value. When examined at the age of 3 years and 10 months the most impressive feature was his severe negativism, which was by no means confined to walking. John, in fact, showed a complete refusal to co-operate in any way and was exceedingly aggressive, the agression being partly directed towards himself in the form of severe head-banging, preferably against somebody else's head, but if not, against the floor or any hard object. He would not co-operate in formal mental testing but he was considered to be functioning at a level corresponding with an I.Q. of about 50, though his potential seemed to be much greater than this and his retardation almost entirely due to the emotional disturbance. John was not typically autistic at this stage but he did have a number of autistic mannerisms and characteristics.

Condition on Admission

Physical examination—John was quite healthy apart from a number of bruises and injuries to his forehead which were self-inflicted. These bruises were of different ages and some in the past had obviously been quite severe. He had an inconstant squint but otherwise there was nothing physically wrong with him. He looked healthy apart from the bruises and slight pallor. He was well cared for but he still wore diapers and was not toilet trained. He was grossly over-active.

Behaviour—John would not let go of his mother and would only walk or stand on his feet when he had finger-tip contact with her. Despite his mother being present, he jumped, rocked,

119

stamped and kept shouting ' Ah '. He was extremely restless and kept trying to tip the chairs over. Whenever he wanted to examine surfaces or ash-trays or other objects, he held mother's hand and pulled her towards them. If he wanted to pick up an object from the floor, he made mother bend down too so that he could reach it while still maintaining contact with her. When frustrated he either banged his head on the ground or on other objects, or he rushed towards bigger objects such as chairs or desks and banged them with his bottom. When he was forcibly separated from his mother, he either went quite rigid, as though in opisthotonos, and banged his head very hard, or he jackknifed and collapsed—even when mother went a few inches away from his finger-tips. His extremely disturbed behaviour had obviously been a great strain on his mother, who was now inclined to take refuge in detachment and disinterest—for example, by putting him in his cot.

Speech—John's speech was obviously retarded in relation to his age; nevertheless, there were certain phrases which showed that his intellectual potential might be considerably higher than his present level of behaviour would indicate. He spoke a monotonous voice, high pitched, whining, and without any variation in tone. Although he could speak appropriately, he kept monotonously repeating certain phrases in a manner which mother found exasperating. For example, ' Want to go to the cot ', ' Want to go to the telephone ', ' Want to go and see Gran '. There were other forms of communication, mostly assertive or angry. For instance, he shouted ' Ah ' when he was annoyed or when he wanted something done. Alternatively, when he was frustrated, he just rushed over and banged a piece of furniture near the person involved.

Responsiveness—Clearly John *could* respond to his mother, to other people and to the reality situation. However, he was so intensely negativistic that his responses mostly took the form of refusal to co-operate, and evident anger. He could respond to all the sensory modalities but he seemed to be impervious to the pain caused by head-banging; he often failed to respond to the spoken word, and he showed occasional characteristic visual avoidance, turning his eyes just to the left of the person who was talking to him. He made no response to other children and only very limited response to adults, apart from his mother. Occasionally he smiled normally, but most of his smiles seemed imitative and conveyed no happiness.

Play and behaviour—John was too distractable and over-active to play properly with anything. He fingered all sorts of objects around the room, tearing at pieces of paper, knocking on ash-trays, fingering everything momentarily and clumsily. When checked in his disruptive behaviour, he became angry and showed the various negativistic responses described above. There were however, no well-developed, clear-cut rituals.

Mood—John was clearly tense and unhappy. The only emotional expression to which he could give vent was rage. Although much of the rage was directed against himself, chiefly in the form of head-banging, he could also express this rage against strangers and his mother. For instance, he tried to dig his nails into people or to pinch them or poke at their eyes or bite them. Mother felt entirely defeated in her attempts to sustain a relationship from which she got no pleasure. She did not hesitate to describe his unsatisfactory behaviour in his presence and John himself repeating ' John's a bad boy ' very frequently.

In four months since admission to hospital, there has been a dramatic change in John's behaviour. At first he continued to bang his head and refused to walk unless one particular nurse was holding his hand. He also showed temper-tantrums and refused to eat, usually scattering his food all over the floor and the other children. At first these symptoms caused almost as much anxiety to the staff as they had done to his mother but his improvement began when an efficient protective head-dress was fitted and the staff were instructed to ignore his head-banging and his tantrums. Coping with his feeding problems was just as difficult. (It will be noted that he had chosen the two symptoms which cause more distress than any others, since they are both injurious to the child.) Luckily, however, the weather was hot and John did not chose to impose upon himself the ultimate punishment, namely, refusal to drink. So, when he was thirsty, he was given no drink except milk or ' Complan ' and in getting enough fluid he also got enough nourishment. The staff were, therefore, able to ignore his refusal to eat and to remove him from the dining room when he began to throw the food about. After a few weeks he was eating quite

121

well. With the improvement in his symptoms his mother was able more easily to accept him during her visits, the length of which could, therefore, slowly be increased. The negativism has diminished considerably and he is beginning to make all-round progress; but, of course, he remains a serious problem.

The cases of John and June are, of course, extreme examples of severe negativism. But negativistic features do, of course, occur in most children; and they are particularly common in severely disturbed children, most of all in autistic children. Indeed, in many cases, it seems that the main obstacle to treatment is the child's need to thwart the parents and other adults by a refusal to co-operate by learning or intellectual effort or by normal and appropriate behaviour.

It is not suggested that there is, in the cases described above, no element of true withdrawal, for, as pointed out above, everyone withdraws to some extent, and these children would be more likely to adopt this mechanism if they were in the habit of assuming the symptom of withdrawal. It is perhaps a question of the conscious level at which the withdrawal takes place. Some autistic infants seem never to have become involved with reality—they cannot be said to withdraw even on an unconscious level. Older children who withdraw do not make a conscious decision to do so; the impulse to withdraw (or the lack of an impulse towards involvement) is an entirely unconscious process. But in these pseudo-schizophrenic children, the withdrawal is almost at conscious level. A child can be truly withdrawn, or he can pretend to take no notice; and these two states are at the opposite ends of a continuum, with all degrees of conscious or unconscious (though purposive) withdrawal in between.

The Ganser syndrome in adults appears to be a kind of hysterical assumption of psychotic illness, the patient ' acts mad ' but his motivation is at an unconscious level. This condition lies between that of the true schizophrenic on the one hand and the malingerer on the other. In the same way, this state of pseudo-schizophrenic negativism may be regarded as lying between that of a child who is pretending to take no notice (or 'acting mad') and that of one who is truly withdrawn or uninvolved. Similarly there is probably a good deal of conscious or semi-conscious exaggeration of psychotic symptoms in children who are truly partially withdrawn, but at the same time involved with reality and with people sufficiently to need to impress them or to influence them.

CHAPTER 8

TREATMENT, EDUCATION AND TRAINING

The treatment and education of autistic children is notoriously difficult. Perhaps this is because it has been hard to understand why they become autistic, for, logically, treatment must be related to causation. One's approach to the child and the methods one employs in treatment and training must, if possible, be based on one's conception of the nature of the disease process. In the absence of clear ideas on causation, our efforts in the past have been largely empirical, and largely ineffectual. Conventional methods of treatment and orthodox methods of teaching have been tried and found wanting; play therapy and psychoanalysis, conditioning techniques and intensive individual teaching have ended very often in discouragement and disillusionment, and as the child fails to improve after endless hours of treatment, the therapist or the teacher, unable to accept this as a failure of his own personality or skill, tends to regard the child as untreatable and unteachable and to turn his attention to less barren fields. The more conscientious or idealistic one is, the more devasting is the effect of the child's failure to respond.

Eventually, efforts at teaching are largely abandoned, and physical methods of treatment are applied—electric shock treatment, tranquillizers, prolonged narcosis, insulin and other endocrine preparations. These may effect some symptomatic improvement, and doctors may be driven to use them because the person who has to look after the child demands that something be done to make him more manageable, less noisy, less self-destructive. But they have not appeared thus far to halt, much less reverse, the disease process, and many of the children deteriorate steadily until they can only be contained in the subnormality hospital or state institution.

It may therefore be appropriate to review our methods of

treatment and education in the light of the foregoing discussions on the nature of autism, and of case histories of children who have improved or have deteriorated. From such a review some general principles can be tentatively suggested.

Early Treatment

We must begin our attempts at treating autistic children as early as possible, for once the autistic way of life has become established for years, or even months, it is exceedingly difficult in the present state of our knowledge to reverse it even partially. Early diagnosis and early treatment are, then, our prime concerns.

Treatment of Physical Ill Health

An attempt must be made to diagnose and treat any underlying physical disability which may be acting as a predisposing or precipitating factor, with the proviso that we must try to avoid making the treatment so unpleasant as to constitute an additional motive for withdrawal. Physical treatment must include an attempt to remedy any metabolic or endocrine dysfunction which may be present, and appropriate physical methods must be employed to improve bodily function. Thus, even with children whose sensory disabilities seem to have a large 'functional' or emotional element, employment of a hearing aid, correction of squint, improvement of gait and posture can be attempted; but carefully, so as not to risk making life so unpleasant as to provoke further withdrawal by the child.

Drug Treatment

The search must be continued for a drug which will improve symptoms. Drugs employed hitherto, even those which are of such great benefit in adult schizophrenics, have been disappointing when used with autistic children, except to relieve symptoms in severely deteriorated cases, in which they have to be used in very large doses. For many years the present writer and his colleagues did try the effect on the autistic children of drugs for which successes were claimed but none of them afforded more than temporary symptomatic relief. Large doses of phenothiazines will sometimes quieten a disturbed child but the effect seems to be lost on prolonged administration. In a few cases, hyperkenetic symptoms have been relieved by amphetamines and these are probably worth trying in all such cases.

It is of interest that the nurses having intimate care of the children usually object to the administration of the ' tranquillizing ' drugs, and it seems that the reason is that they feel the drugs make the children even less accessible. This is not really surprising because the effect of most of these drugs is to render the patient less concerned with reality. What is really needed is not a tranquillizer but a drug which will increase the patient's awareness of the emotional needs of other people and his ability to identify with them and respond to them—a drug which eludes the pharmacologists of today just as the love-potion eluded the alchemists of the middle ages.

Electric Shock Treatment

This does seem to have a definite place in our armamentarium, particularly as a means of cutting short an acutely disturbed episode. As Bender points out, time is short and we must try to avoid the rapid deterioration which tends to occur if such an episode is prolonged. It appears that, in some hands, electric shock treatment is very often helpful, but the course of treatment will often have to be intensive and prolonged. Four or five treatments a week for four or even five weeks may be necessary. It is of course essential that psychotherapeutic measures and individual attention to the child should be increased rather than decreased while EST is being given. The present writer's practice is to employ this treatment only during acutely disturbed phases in older (adolescent) patients.

Psychotherapy

Psychotherapeutic treatment of autistic children involves two mutually dependent processes—*treatment of the family* and *treatment of the child himself.*

Psychotherapy with the Family

Where the mother–child relationship is seriously disturbed, or where there is incompatibility between the child and the rest of the family, or the emotional situation in the family is unsatisfactory, we must endeavour to support, advise and, where necessary, treat the mother and perhaps other members of the family. Whenever possible we will endeavour to treat the child at home, doing our best at out-patients' clinics to relieve any family tensions which may have developed, getting the child into a nursery school or day hospital or training centre or special school, and advising parents and teachers about the child's treatment and training along the lines indicated below. But experience over many years has shown that in the long run most parents have to request the child's admission to hospital for the sake of the rest of the family. Particularly in those cases in which a vicious circle of rejection may have been set up—the child's illness making it more difficult for the family to accept him, so that he tends to withdraw further and become more ill—it will often be advisable to remove the child from the incompatible family situation and place him with another relative, or in hospital.

It is certainly true that, in the present writer's experience, the successful cases have been drawn almost entirely from those in whom the autism was diagnosed early, with early admission to hospital, maintenance of close connections with the family, intensive counselling of parents, and return to the family as soon as possible, with intensive follow-up treatment at out-patients and supervision at school. Here again, however, it must be emphasized that removal from home must be effected in such a way as not to constitute a severe additional emotional trauma. It must be gradual, and complete loss of contact between mother and child is nearly always undesirable. If he has to be admitted to hospital then it is best to arrange for him to be introduced to the hospital by a series of visits of increasing duration. If possible, the mother should be admitted to the hospital with the child and should separate herself from the child only gradually, after he has become accustomed to the group in which he is to live. At Smiths Hospital, Henley on Thames, there is a parents' hostel in which the child can live with his mother—and if necessary the rest of the family too—during the period of the child's introduction to the hospital. At a later time, very regular and increasingly frequent attendance at the hospital by mother is advisable. Usually, however, it is advisable, after the child's slow introduction into the hospital, for him and the mother to have a rest from each other before she begins to visit with increasing frequency. In some cases, the mother–child relationship is so disrupted as to constitute complete rejection on either side. Where this occurs, the relationship may have to be broken physically for the time being and an attempt made to reconstitute it on a different level later on.

Mother Substitutes

Whilst the relationship with the mother is suspended or limited the child must be given an opportunity to make a quasi-maternal relationship with a substitute mother—a relative or a member of the hospital staff. Such relationships are never so intimate as those achieved with the child's own mother, disturbed though this may be, and it is relatively easy to break off such relationships in due course. Some mothers may, not unnaturally, tend to resent the taking over of the child by another woman, even temporarily. This calls for special awareness and special skill on the part of the nurse. All mothers of mentally abnormal or handicapped children tend to feel, often quite illogically and almost completely unconsciously, considerable guilt. Many such mothers torture themselves by trying to find out where they have gone wrong.

Others convert their guilt into feelings of antagonism towards those involved in the care or treatment of the child, and it is always very easy for the mother to justify such antagonism. After all, no-one can love her child like she can, and it is very rarely possible for a nurse in charge of a group of children to give the child the same standard of physical care as can be given by a mother devoting most of her energy and thought to the child. A mother whose whole being has been concentrated on efforts to care for her child may feel terribly at a loss when the child goes into hospital; and if the child happens to improve, her sense of failure or frustration may be all the greater.

Criticism of the hospital is therefore to be expected and experience has shown that the best way of avoiding or mollifying this is to involve the mother very closely in the work of the hospital and the care of her own child, and perhaps of some of the other children also at times, as soon as possible. In this way the mother tends to feel that she is part of a team which is seeking to help her child, and this feeling is increased very greatly if she has frequent contact with other mothers of children in the hospital. Parent groups, therefore, and meetings with nurses, teachers and other members of the staff constitute an exceedingly important part of the treatment programme.

Intensive work by the psychiatrists and psychiatric social workers with the mother, and often the father and sometimes other members of the family, should continue throughout the period of the child's residence in hospital. Supportive work with the mother is one of the most difficult and delicate of the tasks involved in treatment of the child. This is primarily the field of the psychiatric social worker, but the psychiatrist may also have to concentrate his efforts at this point for long periods. The essential task is to try to relieve the mother of her anxiety and to get her to see that her feelings of guilt, though real and understandable, are entirely inappropriate. No word more pejorative than ' incompatability ' should be used, and to talk of coldness or mishandling or over-meticulousness is as inappropriate as it is unwise. Unfortunately, a certain amount of rejection by the mother, conscious or unconscious, is in many cases inevitable, simply because the child's illness involves his effectual rejection of the mother; and the more the mother wants to love the child, the greater is her feeling of frustration when he can give her nothing back. Moreover, the disruption of the family life, which may have been complete in some cases, means that the mother's whole life's work is threatened. It may be ruining her relationships with her husband or the other children, and the mother may for many years have been unable to have any life of her own because of the demands of her autistic child. The desperate distress of the parents has therefore to be understood and their inappropriate feelings of guilt assuaged. Unless this is done the mother's relationship with the child cannot be satisfactorily reconstituted and his progress will be thereby impeded.

In some cases, though by no means all, there is a real emotional disturbance in the mother, which may be obvious but is in some cases deep-seated. Rarely, the mother may be depressed or frankly schizophrenic. More often she is seriously anxious, with perhaps severe, though concealed, personality problems of her own; or she may have problems with her husband or her own mother which are indirectly affecting the child. In such cases, the psychiatrist must recognize and treat the emotional problems in the family. If he fails to do so, the child has little chance of real improvement.

As the mother visits the hospital more frequently, the child is treated to an increasing extent through the mother. The frequency of home visits also is progressively increased and close contact is kept with the family during and after the child's stay in hospital. The hospital staff will involve the mother in their methods of training of the child and hope that these will be continued after he has left the hospital. One of the greatest difficulties here is that the child may refuse to do things for his mother which he is willing to do for other people, and this, of course, is a further source of distress. For this reason it is better that the mother shall not have continuous care of the child throughout the 24 hours, and this, of course, applies to nursing and teaching staff as well. Looking after these children is an excessively demanding task. Unfortunately there are never enough nurses to do it, and one of the great difficulties in running a hospital or school for autistic children is to persuade those who find the money that a very high ratio of staff to patients is necessary.

At all stages it is essential that the mother and the rest of the family should be aware of the level of activities which the child has reached in the hospital. It is essential that when the child is with the mother, either in the ward at the hospital or at home, he must not be allowed to slip back to the level of behaviour he exhibited prior to admission to hospital. For example, if in the hospital he has been taught to dress himself and to do so in a certain routine, it is essential that the mother should not, out of love for the child or the desire to get him dressed quickly, dress him herself. Similarly, with regard to feeding; if he has been taught to feed himself with a knife and fork he must not be allowed to go back to a spoon and pusher or to feeding himself with his fingers. If he is not allowed to jump from the table whilst the meal is in progress in the hospital, it is important that he should not be allowed to do so at home. If in the hospital he is not allowed to play with pieces of plastic tape or leaves cut off trees, it is essential that he should not be allowed to do this at home either. In the hospital he only gets his breakfast after he has done his morning 'chores', say, going to the toilet, washing himself, dressing himself and sweeping round his bed. It is important that the same routine and the same reward should be insisted upon at home.

The difficulty, of course, is to persuade mother that assisting the child and indulging his desire to escape into mannerisms or regress into an infantile mode of behaviour is, in fact, preventing him from making progress. Because of the guilt which the mother feels over the child's illness, and because of her love for him, she tends to do things for him which he can perfectly well do for himself. Once he has learned to lace his shoes no one should ever lace them for him again. To ensure the acceptance of this principle and practice by the parents is, paradoxically, one of the most difficult tasks of the nursing staff and the social worker. Apparently the mother feels that she must be able to do more for her child than the hospital can. There is, moreover, a tendency in some mothers to despair. The mother of one severely autistic seven-year-old boy was asked whether she still tried to train him to the pot. She replied, ' No. They do try to teach him at the training centre but at home I have just given up and I clean him up when he dirties himself. I suppose I feel that is the least I can do for him.' Once the mother has sunk into this kind of despairing attitude, it is exceedingly difficult to give her the necessary encouragement to emerge from it. She may even resent the fact that the hospital has been able to make progress with the child and to teach him skills which he has not learned under her care. This is unfortunate, but very easily understandable as one talks to the mothers and appreciates how desperately they have tried and how bitter is their sense of failure. In many cases the father or other members of the family are even more difficult to convince than mother that there is some hope that the child may improve. In some cases there is resistance to the idea that the child can make progress, because the family have tried so often and so hard and been so disappointed at the failure to make progress that, by the time the child comes into hospital, they have had enough of it and cannot bear any longer to continue to attempt an apparently hopeless and humiliating task. Some parents (and even some nurses and social workers and psychiatrists) have to take refuge in a conviction that the child is suffering from an irreversible ' organic ' disease simply because they cannot bear the affront to their own self-respect which they feel to be implied if the child fails to make progress in their hands. Even in these cases, however, one can insist that, whatever the cause of the child's disability, attempts must be made to improve his mode of behaviour, and this can only be done by adoption of a consistent, progressive policy of treatment and training by hospital, school and home. After the child leaves the hospital and returns to live at home (assuming sufficient improvement has taken place to make this possible) and in those cases in which it seems advisable that the child should remain at home, the assiduous supportive work with the family must continue. It is also necessary to keep in close touch with teachers who have care of the child, and it is essential to enlist the help of the family doctor—otherwise we may find that they and the psychiatrist may be pursuing divergent or incompatible lines of treatment, thus increasing the parental perplexity which we must, at all costs, seek to avoid.

Pre-school Training

The first step must be to attempt to give the child pre-school training. If the child has not been admitted to hospital this stage of training will have to be carried out in a nursery school or a junior training centre, or perhaps even in a special care unit, depending on the child's age and the severity of his illness. There have been a few successful examples of parents banding together to provide their own pre-school training unit for autistic children but, in this country, such initiative is only feasible in large centres of population, and only necessary until the local authority is able to provide the necessary facilities. It is essential that pre-school training be instituted as soon as possible and interrupted as seldom as possible, even though the child appears to make no response for long periods; for experience has shown that even during such periods the child may be learning a great deal more than is apparent at the time. The work of the mother, the nurse, the teacher, the psychologist, the psychiatric social worker and the doctor is intimately related and the very closest co-operation is necessary throughout.

As far as children in hospital are concerned, of course, it is not essential that this initial training of the child should be done only by nurses; indeed, there is some indication that the nurses' training and approach to the patient is not ideal for this work of pre-school teaching and training. In the general wards of a hospital, the nurse is trained to cosset and protect. When the patient is ready to start helping himself he is placed more and more in the care of others, such as occupational therapists and physiotherapists. The training of the psychiatric nurse has been affected by this tradition; she too has been trained to cosset, to comfort and protect. She has not been trained, or at least not adequately trained in most cases, to stimulate, to occupy, to train, to teach the patient how to live. So there is a danger that the nurse in charge of a group of autistic children may care beautifully for their bodies and their cleanliness and their clothes, but leave their training to someone else, or, alas, to nobody. Yet the nurse is the mother-substitute in hospital; and it is the mother who normally initiates the child's training and education. The psychiatric nurse must be taught to do this work, learning from the psychiatrist, the psychologist, the teacher and the occupational therapist. It is she who has the most opportunity, since like the mother in the home she is with the child most of the day. Moreover, she does not have the week-end off as teachers do, nor does she have the very long school holidays; and it is a fact that these long school holidays are disastrous for the psychotic child's training, whatever their effect on the normal child's education. The nurses are there all the time, and they must be taught how to continue (or initiate) the child's education or occupation or training while the rest of the staff is away. If nurses are not available, then specially trained child-care workers must be employed, as is increasingly the practice in the U.S.A.

The Beginnings of Education

Making a Relationship

The basic principle in training and education of autistic children is that the nurse or teacher will first make some sort of relationship with the child, using whatever activity the child will undertake as a bridge between them, and trying to cajole him into gradually expanding his aimless and often manneristic activity into something which begins to approach a purposive and, eventually, an educational pursuit or skill.

It has been suggested above that in all the cases of childhood autism which the writer has seen, there has been a defect in the relationship between the child and his mother or mother-substitute. Since the child's ability to involve himself with other human beings depends very largely on the success of his initial involvement with mother or mother-substitute, and since every successful relationship encourages the child to form further and deeper relationships, it is evident that the first essential step in treatment is that the mother-figure shall form a real relationship with the child and he with her. We therefore have to give both mother and child every help in making or restoring their relationship. Usually, by the time the child is brought for treatment, his inability to relate to her (however it may have been caused in the first place) has meant that the mother gets no ' feed-back ', no reward, in her attempt to love him. Because she gets no response from him, her inclination to continue her attempts to love him slowly becomes weakened. One cannot go on forever trying to love someone who cannot return one's love. Thus the mother's involvement with the child is diminished; and if the child is getting less from the mother, then his response to her is even further lessened. So the vicious circle is set up and in the worst cases one finds, not merely a failure of positive relationship, but an active rejection on one side or even on both.

If a child has not learned to relate to his mother, then of course his ability to relate to other human beings will be

135

impaired. Worse than this—if the child cannot make a satisfactory relationship with his mother, he tends to resent her relationships with other people, particularly his brothers or sisters; and if he cannot get the real deep affection which he needs from mother, then at least he tries to monopolize her attention and time at the expense of any other people with claims on her, and he very rapidly becomes over-demanding as well as fundamentally withdrawn. So we have a child who is unable to make a proper relationship with mother; who, therefore, cannot relate to other human beings, particularly children; and who, in fact, tends to resent any time or attention given by mother to other members of the family. They in turn fail to form a warm relationship with the child, or may even reject him, and this causes a further impairment in the child's ability to make relationships with other human beings. The first task in treatment, therefore, must be to make a relationship, somehow or other, with the child. To do this one has to be prepared to devote unbroken periods of time exclusively to him. All other interests and persons must be set aside during these periods and it is much better to devote a comparatively short period of time exclusively to the child than to try to look after him and another child at the same time or to pursue an activity—such as housework—in which the child is not interested.

The next problem is: what activities should one attempt to pursue with the patient? Obviously, one wishes to divert his energy and interest from his aimless pursuits and mannerisms and stereotyped behaviour into some activity which is purposeful and, if possible, useful or educational, or, at least, acceptable. At first this often seems an impossible task, for the child declines to interest himself in anything except his mannerisms. He may resist by tantrums or by attempted flight, by becoming temporarily ' blind ' or ' deaf ' through visual or auditory avoidance, by becoming ' jelly-fingered ' or ' jelly-legged ', or by such tricks as screaming or urinating or defaecating a little bit all the time so as to preclude useful activity on the part of the adult.

Usually, one has to seize an activity in which the child is already interested, in however rudimentary a way, and try to expand around this. For example, there are some autistic children in whom ' rocking ' is the dominant and almost exclusive activity. If all else fails one must be prepared to rock with the child; then to rock with him in one's arms; then on to a rocking chair; then on to a see-saw; then on to a swing; then on to a climbing rope or frame; and perhaps on to a trampoline; then into more generalized romping play in the garden or, ideally, a large playroom with plenty of sturdy equipment in it. All the time the adult will share in the child's activity, feeling his way carefully and not pushing the child into activities which may be frightening or too violent for the time being. Where this is being attempted in the home, it is of course very much more difficult because of mother's other preoccupations—for example, she has to get the housework done. But even here something can be done to involve the child with the mother's activities and vice versa. For example, most children like playing with water; even more, they like playing with water containing suds or detergents. Supposing mother does the washing-up and the child stands on a chair beside her at the sink playing with the suds and a dishmop; it may be possible in these circumstances to guide his hands in helping mother to wash a plate, and then putting the plate in the rack. Then, perhaps, the child can be induced to wash two or three plates whilst mother stands beside him admiring him and mixing the purposeful activity with play. Of course mother must make the activity seem more like play than work; and she must not let it appear to the child that she is anxious to get him to carry out the activity—otherwise the negativism which may be such a strong element in the child's disability will prevent him from joining in.

Slowly, the washing-up activity can be expanded to include

clearing the table and putting the crockery away after washing. The activity has to be very slowly extended at both ends, in the hope of increasing the child's span of attention, which is characteristically short for his age. If the child is being looked after at home, these household chores are probably a better way of getting the child's attention and interest than activities like drawing and painting, though these, too, have their place. Cooking also is surprisingly successful with autistic children. One begins with playing with dough (and this is a very suitable plaything since, unlike many other materials, it does not matter if it gets eaten). Then one can proceed to rolling or shaping the dough and eventually to putting it in the oven and—most important of all—taking it out and eating it. Consuming the product is the reward of the completed activity and this is what makes cooking so valuable.

Conditioning Procedures

These are having an increasing vogue at the present time, but it must be emphasized that they do not involve any new fundamental concept. Indeed, it can be said that all training is built up on a series of conditioning procedures. The principle is basically the simple one, that acceptable behaviour is always immediately rewarded, and unacceptable behaviour is always immediately punished. These, of course, have been the principles of training animals since time immemorial, and they have also been used, with modifications, in the training of human beings. With the higher animals, particularly dogs and anthropoids, it is possible to obtain the required response by giving, on the completion of the required activity, not the immediate reward but a signal, or even a complicated series of signals, which the animal knows will eventually culminate in the presentation of the reward. At its highest level, in human beings, the response can be obtained merely by promising the individual that a reward will follow upon completion of the activity;

or, conversely, that punishment will follow if the activity is not satisfactorily completed. This process, of course, breaks down in the autistic child because he is liable not to listen to the promise or threat; or because he is able to ignore or 'disassociate' the reward or punishment. If he is so withdrawn as to be uninterested in the reward and its implications, and if he is able to 'shut off' the painful stimulus of the punishment then, of course, he is unlikely to respond. There is a further incentive which we use in training animals: it involves getting the animal to 'love' the trainer, so that he will carry out an activity in response to an order from his trainer though not from anyone else—the 'reward', of course, consisting merely of a pat or some shared activity with his beloved. The extent to which this incentive operates varies with the species; it is very high in dogs, and in human beings it is probably the most important single motivating factor. Mostly, as Freud pointed out, we do things for love.

Here again, however, the autistic misses out; he does not really love anybody to the normal degree, so he is not interested in doing things to please other people; therefore this very valuable incentive is lacking, even as an adjunct in getting him to perform activities which will be rewarded.

Basically it is these factors which make it difficult to teach or train autistic children and, as might be expected, conditioning procedures have severe limitations when applied to them. However, there is no doubt that they can be trained to do puzzles or match colours or to do simple self-care activities, or even to speak, by using these techniques. The trouble is, unfortunately, that in themselves these skills mean nothing. It is only if they form a bridge between the child and some other human being, or if they get him more interested in reality as a whole, that they are capable of being expanded into further activities as part of a more normal way of life. Moreover, the disincentives available are very limited. In certain centres in the United States, for example, electric shocks were used as punishments for

139

unsatisfactory behaviour. Less scientifically minded persons have used beating as the disincentive, or cold baths or ' no dinner '; but in all these methods it is very difficult to decide where the scientific procedure ends and the cruelty begins. Moreover, such cruelty always bestializes the environment; in any case the autistic child soon learns to ' dissociate ' or to become innured to the pain involved in the punishment (his tendency to ' withdrawal ' being thereby reinforced). In the writer's opinion cruelty, however disguised, has no place in the treatment or training of the autistic—or any other—child.

Nevertheless, it is possible to train these children to some extent by *immediate* reward of satisfactory behaviour. One does not threaten or promise, one simply creates a pleasant feeling-tone by presentation of the reward immediately the activity has been carried out, so that the patient associates the carrying out of that activity with a pleasant feeling-tone. In general there are three types of reward which may be used; first, the immediate reward of a pleasant sensation like a grape or a sweet or being thrown up in the air or bounced on the trampoline or taken for a ride; second, the reward of satisfaction in the exercise of a learned skill; and third— we hope—the pleasure of a pat or a hug or a kiss or a word of approbation from another human being *with whom some relationship, however slight, has been achieved through the sharing of activity*. This latter will only supervene after much hard work, and then only if the adult conceives some real affection for the child; but it is, of course, far and away the most important object of the whole technique, because once the child has begun to be motivated even partially by some kind of attachment, however minimal, to another human being, then he is starting on the way to recovery.

Obviously, conditioning procedures have to be used at all stages and the principle of never rewarding an unaccept- able activity but always rewarding the acceptable activity has to be closely followed. It is, of course, best not to *promise* the reward, because if one does so the child is liable to refuse both the activity and the reward—as much as to say ' I am not going to be bought or bent to your will by bribes—I would much rather go without the reward '. So the reward has to be carefully chosen and, as a rule, unobtrusively given.

Possibly even more important than the regular rewarding of acceptable behaviour is the avoidance of rewarding unacceptable activities. If the mother reacts to the child's rocking or soiling or masturbation by becoming distressed or angry, then this, paradoxically, may constitute a reward in itself, for not only does it fix mother's attention and interest but also it provokes a reaction from her which the child's negavitism may welcome. On such occasions the adult has to react as far as possible by ignoral or subtly altering the focus of his attention. For example, there was one child at the hospital who could not go home because whenever she did so she continually leaked faeces all over the house. If a diaper was put on she removed it and continued to destroy the family's furnishings and their equanimity with this peculiarly distressing habit. The child's reward in this case was the extreme distress of mother and the diversion of her attention from the younger sibling. Mother was being punished for her rejection of the child but of course her rejection was very much increased by the child's method of punishing and provoking her. At the hospital the child did not behave in this way because there was no emotional response and the child did not enjoy being bathed and then put out in the garden. If mother left the baby at home and came to visit our patient in the parents' hostel, giving her whole time and attention to the patient, then, of course, the soiling did not occur.

Using the Child's Rituals

One of the features of the behaviour of seriously disturbed and autistic children is the tendency to impose rituals on themselves and the people around them. As suggested above, this seems to be a protective mechanism against an unpredictable and, therefore, a disturbing or frightening environment. This need for an established ritual has to be used in occupying and training the autistic child. The principle is that the child will follow the same schedule of behaviour every day but that the schedule should be slowly but continuously extended and expanded, thus leaving less and less time for unsatisfactory behaviour and psychotic mannerisms. In fact, of course, the patient only indulges in his mannerisms and stereotyped behaviour ' Faute de mieux '; he would just as soon bounce on the trampoline as stand and rock. He would just as soon play with the dough as with faeces. In the hospital it is possible to get the children together in the gymnasium and encourage them to complete a simple obstacle course; or to roller-skate; or hit a ball; and there are similar skills he can be taught in the house and garden.

Once he has learned a skilled activity he will, for a time at any rate, get some pleasure out of pursuing it (this is to be seen in those autistic children who, without instruction, learn some complicated activity like spinning various objects or prising tiles out of walls). He will then pursue the activity *for its own sake*. (Experience with teaching-machines has shown that one of the most effective incentives for autistic children, as for normal children, is the pleasure they derive from exercising a learned skill.) We must make the maximum use of this kind of incentive.

Habit Training

So we try to get the child involved in a progressively expanding routine of continual training. For example, the patient gets up in the morning, and goes straight to the W.C.; then under the shower, which mother has turned on and adjusted for him (but later he will learn to adjust the temperature of the water himself); then he dries himself (with mother's assistance as necessary) and then makes his bed, again with mother's help. Then he goes downstairs and lays the table whilst mother is getting the breakfast. *Immediate* provision of the breakfast he likes is the reward for completing the first few tasks of the morning. All this sounds so obvious and simple that it seems hardly worth describing. Yet it probably involves mother in careful preparation the previous night, in her getting up much earlier than would otherwise be necessary, and in the husband assuming the care of the other child or children during this particular period of the day. It also involves the mother in endlessly patient repetition and quiet insistence on the morning routine. But the autistic child can be taught, just as an ordinary infant can be taught. The only difference is that it requires infinitely more time and patience, and persistence. It is, of course, very much quicker and easier to do these things for the child than to teach him to do them himself; but once he has learned his routine he may be content to pursue it, leaving the mother freedom to look after the rest of the family at that time, so that she will be able to give individual attention to the autistic child in teaching him a new task later in the day.

The same principle, of course, applies to nurses who are looking after a group of children in hospital or training centre. The process is exactly the same as the ' habit-training ' which was introduced into the chronic wards of the old mental hospitals, effecting such a remarkable change in the physical and emotional atmosphere of the ward and the morale of the patients. Each patient is taught one section of the routine at a time, the nurses concentrating attention on this patient until he has become reliable. Then they concentrate on the next patient, and so on, until the whole group is involved in the routine. With the autistic children this kind of training is applied not only to the toilet and to self-care but to an expanding range of activities, which, in time, occupies a considerable portion of the day, leaving the nurse free to introduce a new patient into the routine and give him the individual training which is essential in the early stages.

Not only does this method enable the nurse (or the mother) to cope with several children at the same time, and even to get on with some of her household management whilst the children are engaged upon their routine occupations, but it also involves the children functioning as part of a group. Into such a group shared activities can eventually be introduced, although this further step requires great skill and patience on the part of the adult. The great skill, of course, lies in getting the child to regard the activities as play, rather than ' chores ', in the first instance, and in rewarding the child perhaps without his realizing that he is being rewarded for the completion of the task.

Needless to say, one person cannot continue to cajole and supervise the child in its routine activities throughout the day. One of the difficulties that the mothers of these children face is that the child requires constant attention for eighteen hours a day, every single day of the week. One cannot imagine anything more likely to provoke eventual rejection of the child than such a situation. It is, therefore, absolutely essential that there should be more than one person looking after the child. A play-group, a training centre, a day hospital or a school must therefore be found for the child, and he should begin to attend the group very early. Even at three years the mother is probably going to need to have the child in other hands during a proportion of the day. And all the time, of course, the mother or the nurse or the teacher needs constant support and encouragement; for they are attempting what must surely be the most difficult job in the world—to teach the unteachable, to make a relationship with, and secure the interest of, the child who has ' opted out ' and literally does not ' want to know '. Such is the frustration which can be caused by endless and apparently unrewarded attempts to train these patients that an attitude of despair tends eventually to creep in, even in the most determined and devoted mother or nurse. It is perhaps for this reason that those concerned with looking after these children so often turn to theories of 'organicity', of inevitability and essential ineducability. Sometimes the task is so onerous that the human being faced with it simply has to find an escape. Eventually, in some cases, one has to accept that there are tasks too heavy for us to cope with satisfactorily in the present state of our knowledge, and one has to be contented with small gains and limited objectives. Nevertheless, in every single case *something* can be done to get the child nearer to a degree of independence and a reasonably normal way of life.

Group Activities—Sharing

Autistic children do not make adequate relationships with adults and even less so with other children, whom they do not distinguish for practical purposes from other objects in their environment. Thus they tend to walk 'through' or 'over' them, rather than around them. A photograph of a group of autistic children will invariably show them in self-imposed isolation. However, if the adult in charge of a group of autistics is seen to give attention to one of the children, then the others will tend to intrude. If the adult then turns to the intruder, the first child may resist in order to retain the adult's attention or he may then withdraw more completely, thus breaking for the time being the tenuous relationship that he has with the adult. The only way to deal with this in the first instance is to make sure of devoting a part of each day to giving the child undivided attention. Our patients cannot tolerate triangular, much less quadrangular, situations or relationships. They have to have a one-to-one relationship and to become secure in this relationship before they can tolerate sharing the adult even momentarily with another child. Once they have a firm base in the acceptance by one adult they may have some ability to go forward and make relationships with others. But they will only do so gingerly and for very short periods at first. On the other hand some progress

145

can be made through shared activities, for example, the see-saw which will not operate unless there is somebody sitting on the other end. Splashing games in the pool also need the co-operation of another human being. So do games like ' ring-o'-roses ' or ' oranges-and-lemons '. Once a child has learned to kick a football and begins to enjoy doing so he needs another human being to kick it back to him. From this, by very gradual stages, we would hope, over a very long period, to build up to the point where the child was capable of playing a very elementary game of football— with, necessarily, some association with the other players. It seems we have to go back to the infantile situation wherein the child has the monopoly of his mother's attention and try to make him so secure in his early relationship with one person, and then with a succession of undemanding and uncompetitive human beings, that he will feel secure enough to venture into the real world and its relationships.

All these children have an interest, often a distressingly exclusive interest, in their own bodies. We must try to show the child how to find new and satisfying uses for his body. We have to use the exhilaration of chasing as an introduction to racing, for example, and thus introduce an element of competition which necessarily involves some recognition of the existence *and the uses* of other children. A recurrent problem is the child's tendency to ' stick ' at a certain level. It may, for example, be extremely difficult to get him to progress beyond the stage of jig-saw puzzles and for a long time the only advance he will make is to do bigger and better and more complicated puzzles at increased speeds. This, of course, is comparable with the tendency of many normal children to ' stick ' at certain levels—a tendency which tests the skill and ingenuity of all teachers. Every child, including the autistic child, needs an individual approach. One may be able to expand the interest in jig-saw puzzles into a game involving finding the missing pieces of the puzzle hidden in various places in the room, or we can persuade him to attempt cut-outs, stencils, painting the pieces of a jigsaw to make a pattern and perhaps, in the end, fret-sawing the pieces. Here again, perhaps at this stage an element of competition with another child can be introduced, or the way may lie through other games involving the fitting of shapes, perhaps in the use of constructional toys. Anything the child will or can do must be a step towards further activity, and the teacher or nurse will be prepared to switch to an entirely different field of activity if a complete block is reached for the time being on a previously profitable line. If the child will sing but not talk, we can teach him through song; if he will only scribble, we can encourage him to finger-paint. Perhaps we can introduce him to clay modelling only by letting him throw clay at the walls; but we must never let him get stuck at scribbling or finger-painting, or throwing clay, even if we have to guide his hand gently into a more progressive activity.

In the play-group or the training centre the child may consent to be taught skills which seemed beyond him at home; and, conversely, sometimes the child will do nothing for the teacher but will do what the teacher has been showing him when he gets back to his mother or the nurse in the evening or at the week-end, or vice versa. One of the difficulties is that there are optimum ages for the acquiring of certain skills and once the child has passed this optimum age it becomes progressively more difficult to teach him the particular skill involved. In these cases one simply has to resign oneself to making the best use of what potential skill remains.

There is, of course, nothing new in most of this; it is part of the basic and enduring philosophy of education. But it is hard indeed to apply it in the case of the autistic child, the child who has ‘ opted out ’, who simply ‘ doesn’t want to know ’, who literally ‘ couldn’t care less ’. The nurse, or the teacher, or the occupational therapist, or the house parent, needs enormous patience, quiet firmness, the ability to use subtle inducements, immediate rewards and, rarely, minor punishments. If she is too strict with the child, he will defeat her by withdrawing further. If she is too permissive, he will do nothing. He must be both cajoled and stimulated. These children will often make sudden advances when excited or angry, but when the situation becomes dangerous or threatening, when people shout in anger or smack them or desert them, the children will often withdraw further than ever.

At first the child will probably only respond to a one-to-one relationship in training or teaching, but as soon as possible he must be introduced into a small group and persuaded to conform to a rudimentary programme or schedule. Once this is established the child will feel more protected and secure and will find it easier to co-operate; for the unpredictability of reality is one of its most frightening aspects, from which these children protect themselves by obsessions and rituals. The firm framework, based on a regular schedule, makes the child's rituals unnecessary. In a predictable environment, he has more confidence and can devote more of his attention to the task in hand and less to warding off reality.

One of the teacher's problems is to know when she must indulgently tolerate the child's obsessions and repetitive questions and when she can safely ignore them or break them. She will be unable to do so until they become *unnecessary* because of the security conveyed by the regular schedule and the teacher's reliable and predictable responses. Group activities on a regular basis, shared treats and trips and jokes—these become the basis of an increasing identification with the group and improve relations with the other children.

Communication

Perhaps the greatest problem of all is that of getting the children to speak. It has long been realized that the prognosis for children who are not speaking at the age of $4\frac{1}{2}$ or 5 years is very much worse than for those who will say even a few words. Therefore, we make enormous efforts to get the children to speak; and perhaps these efforts themselves are the greatest obstacle to success, since in the field of communication, more than any other, the negativism which most of the children show to a greater or lesser extent may be almost impossible to combat. Certainly the old technique of asking the child to repeat odd words or phrases pays no dividends at all, except to increase the child's resistance to speaking. What has to be emphasized is that we are dealing with disinclination, rather than inability, to speak, although, of course, the child who has not learned to speak at the appropriate time will have more difficulty in learning to speak later on, even if he wants to—just as it is more difficult to learn to skate or swim at sixty than at six. But there is no doubt that most of these children *can* speak, and many autistic children who are habitually mute do occasionally speak—for example, when they think no one can hear them (as in bed at night). Sometimes one can get speech from the child which is not used for communication, but seems to be rather an exercise in bodily function, like rocking or running up and down or hopping; and sometimes they can be persuaded to sing words of songs even when they will not speak. They are most likely to utter words or even whole phrases or sentences at moments of great surprise or excitement or anger.

Rage Reduction

Hitherto it has not seemed possible to use these phenomena as a progressive technique in teaching the children to speak. However, a method introduced by Zazlow seems to have possibilities. Zazlow (Zazlow, 1969) (Allen, 1969) calls the treatment ' rage reduction ' and his reasons for adopting this name, together with the rationale on which he bases his approach, are somewhat controversial; but it does seem that the method has great possibilities. Essentially it consists of holding the child, talking to him, manipulating his lips and limbs and so eventually *provoking* (although Zazlow would not use this word) an enraged reaction from the child. This rage reaction is then reduced by dint of continuing

149

to hold the child, with such assistance as may be necessary, until gradually or suddenly the resistance subsides and the child becomes relaxed and calm. Whatever the explanation of this phenomenon (whether it be due to the patient's having so fully given vent to his underlying rage that he has no more to express for the time being; or whether it is due to temporary exhaustion; or to a feeling that attempts to escape are hopeless) the subsequent effect on the child is certainly to make him calmer and more co-operative. It may be that the essential feature is the ' forced ' relationship, the child having no escape from an intimate physical contact with the adult in spite of his tremendous protests; and presumably even the severely autistic child must in these circumstances also be making some kind of emotional contact. What is particularly interesting is that the child shows no disposition to be afraid of, or to avoid, the therapist at subsequent meetings. In between sessions there is a definite improvement, in some cases at any rate. During the treatment sessions some of the children *can* be provoked in their rage to vocalize and often to speak much more than they usually do. What is not yet clear is whether this improvement continues after the series of treatment sessions are terminated, or whether these sessions have to be continued indefinitely, or for a very long period, if real improvement is to be maintained.

The sudden ' capitulation ' of the child during these so-called rage-reduction sessions can be very dramatic. In some ways the process seems to be analogous to the capitulation of the female to the overpowering male in a forced sexual situation—following which some kind of accepting or ambivalent relationship between the man and the woman may continue.

Needless to say, even this method is not entirely new, since it has long been apparent that, as a rule, the best way of dealing with an autistic child in one of the frantic screaming or self-destructive or terror-stricken attacks to which they are prone is to hold the child quite firmly, talking gently to him, until the paroxysm has passed—even if this takes hours or days. Unfortunately, it is very rarely that this can be done, owing to lack of staff time. Parents instinctively resort to this method with their normal children; but they can very rarely sustain it in the extremely harrowing attacks suffered by their autistic children. As a rule the children will vocalize more than usual at these times but what they say tends to be repetitive and, to our ears, nonsensical.

Other methods of teaching children to talk have been disappointing. Conditioning techniques, as described above, have been used and with some success. Unfortunately, the children tend to relapse after a series of treatment sessions is finished and one is left with the impression that the improvement has been due to the intense interest and effort of the therapist which succeeds in making a partial relationship with the child. It is worth having a tape recorder to use during speech-therapy sessions so that the child can hear his own vocalizations, but here again the child tends to lose interest in the tape recorder after a time. What is particularly disappointing is that a child who is almost mute may learn— apparently spontaneously—to say a whole phrase and to use it a good deal for a time, only to lose it slowly or suddenly after a short while. On the other hand it is by no means unknown for an autistic adolescent to begin to say a few words after years of silence, but the words, in these cases, are usually few and far between and poorly articulated.

In the absence of reliable techniques for producing speech we can only continue to use the method of speaking to the child all the time one is alone with him, describing everything that he does, and never demanding a reply.

Schooling

It is almost certainly a mistake to maintain schools exclusively for autistic children. They must have other children with whom they can learn to relate, so they must not be surrounded only by other autistic children. They will not

Conclusion

Conclusion

attempt to communicate with other children who do not themselves communicate. One cannot learn to talk or listen to speech if there is nobody to talk to. Experience has shown that these children do best in units in which there are other kinds of mentally retarded or emotionally disturbed children in roughly equal numbers. Schools for such children must have a high ratio of teachers to children. The methods must be flexible but all the time the aim must be to get the child to accept a regular, ordered and progressive programme.

As soon as possible the child is cautiously and gradually introduced into a normal school. He will nearly always be functioning at well below the normal standard for his age, but it is better for him to be with children of his own age group or a year or so younger. In cases who have to be admitted to hospital, the aim is to have the child attending an ordinary school or an E.S.N. school (if one is available) full time for at least a term before he returns to live at home. In some cases, however, the child may be ready for whole time schooling but not ready to live entirely at home, and in these cases a residential school may be the best placement. Whether the child is living at home or in hospital, it is probably better to introduce him to the school for one or two half days a week at the commencement, and slowly to increase the frequency and duration of his attendance. His introduction into, and maintenance in, a normal school is a matter of the very greatest difficulty, requiring patience, tolerance and devotion on all sides. Not all head teachers are able to tolerate these children in their schools, particularly when classes are large, because of the great amount of individual attention they require. The needs of the normal children cannot be indefinitely subordinated to those of the disturbed. But if the head teacher knows that the hospital or clinic is ready to take over again at short notice, and if the medical side goes to great pains to maintain communications, then the school is likely to be willing to give the child another chance later on.

In all cases it is absolutely essential for the psychiatric team to maintain close contact with the teachers in the school. Continuing contact with the home will, of course, also be necessary, probably throughout the child's adolescence.

Other Forms of Training

At the present stage of our knowledge and skill there will remain a large proportion of cases in which rehabilitation into normal school and family life is not possible; and such children may have to remain in hospital, although an increasing number of them are now able to live at home and attend training centres for the subnormal. Even in those cases in which rehabilitation is not possible, an attempt must be made to give the child as much training as he is capable of absorbing and as much individual care as possible. In this way, even though we may not be able to produce much improvement, we can at least prevent a good deal of the deterioration which occurs in most untreated cases. Very often such patients become stabilized after puberty as medium grade subnormal persons, able to live tolerably happy lives at home or in hospital. As a rule, the psychotic illness tends to burn itself out in early adult life, and at this time further efforts at rehabilitation must be made. The patient must be trained and encouraged to use to the full what physical and mental resources he still retains. Training and retraining must be a continuous and unrelenting process.

When all is said, we know but little about autistic children, and a life-time of experience with them is enough to bring humility to the most arrogant. Our efforts to learn more about them must be continued in great earnestness, not only because of our feeling that many of them, with better luck, might have become very special human beings; but also because, through studying their disabilities, we may stumble upon principles of general application in the field of the development of human abilities and human personality.

REFERENCES

Adams, H. M. and Glasner, P. J. (1954). 'Emotional Involvements in Some Forms of Mutism.' *J. Speech Hear. Disorders*, **19**, 59–69.

Allen, J. (1969). Personal communication.

Arieti, S. (1959). *American Handbook of Psychiatry*, p. 471. New York; Basic Books.

Bannister D. (1968). Brit. Journ. Psychiat. 181. 114. 507.

Basowitz, H., Persky, H., Korchin, S. J. and Grinker, I. G. (1955). *Anxiety and Stress*. Chicago; McGraw-Hill.

Bender, L. and Nichtern, S. (1956). 'Chemotherapy in Child Psychiatry.' *N.Y.S. J. Med.*, **56**, 2791–2795.

— Faretra, G. and Cobrinik, L. (1963). *Recent Advances in Biological Psychiatry*, Vol. 5. New York; Plenum Press.

Bennett, E. L., Diamond, M. C., Kreech, D., and Rosenzweig, M. R. (1964). Environmental determinants of acetylcholinesterase and cholinesterase activities in rat brain. *Science*, 146, 610.

Bleuler, E. (1952). *Dementia Praecox or the Group of Schizophrenias*. (Translated by Joseph Zinkin.) New York; International University Press.

Bowlby, J. (1951). *Maternal Care and Mental Health*. Geneva; W.H.O.

Brune, G. G. and Himwich, H. E. (1963). *Recent Advances in Biological Psychiatry*, Vol. 5, p. 44. New York; Plenum Press.

Cragg, B. G. (1967). Changes in visual cortex on first exposure of rats to light. *Nature*, 215, 5098.

Creak, M. (1951). 'Psychoses in Childhood.' *J. ment. Sci.*, **97**, 545–554.

— (1952). 'Discussion: Psychoses in Childhood.' *Proc. R. Soc. Med.*, **45**, 797–800.

— (1961). (Chairman.) 'The Schizophrenic Syndrome in Childhood. Progress Report of a Working Party.' *Br. med. J.*, **2**, 889–890.

— (1963). 'Childhood Psychosis, A Review of 100 Cases.' *Br. J. Psychiat.*, **109**, 84–89.

— and Ini, S. (1960). 'Families of Psychotic Children.' In *Child Psychology and Psychiatry*, Vol. 1, pp. 156–175. London; Pergamon Press.

Daniels, W. A. (1941). 'A Study of Insulin Tolerance and Glucose Tolerance Tests on Normal Infants.' *J. Paediat.*, **19**, 789.

Despert, J. L. (1947). 'The Early Recognition of Childhood Schizophrenia.' *Med. Clins N. Am.*, **31**, 680–687.

REFERENCES

Faretra, G. and Bender, L. (1964). 'Autonomic Nervous System Responses in Hospitalised Children Treated with LSD and UML.' In *Recent Advances in Biological Psychiatry*, Vol. 7. New York; Plenum Press.

Fenichel, C. (1963). 'Educating the Severely Disturbed Child.' *Pathways in Child Guidance*, 5, March.

Fish, B. (1960). 'Involvement of the Central Nervous System in Infants with Schizophrenia.' *A.M.A. Archs Neurol. Chicago*, **2**, 115–121.

Friedhoff, A. J. and van Winkle, E. (1962). 'The Characteristics of an Amine Found in the Urine of Schizophrenic Patients.' *J. nerv. ment. Dis.*, **135**, 550–555.

Gjessing, R. (1938). 'Disturbance of Somatic Function in Catatonic Periodic Courses and their Compensation.' *J. ment. Sci.*, **84**, 608.

— (1939). *Arch. Psychiat. Nervkrankh.*, **109**, 525.

Goldfarb, W. (1961). *Childhood Schizophrenia*. Cambridge, Mass.; Harvard University Press.

— (1964). 'An Investigation of Childhood Schizophrenia.' *Archs Gen. Psychiatry*, **2**, 620–634.

Grey-Walter, W. (1964). 'Report on Neurophysiological Correlates of Apparent Defects of Sensori-motor Integration in Autistic Children.' Mental Health Research Fund.

Heller, T. (1930). 'Uber Dementia Infantilis.' *Z. Kinderforsch.*, **73**, 611. Translated by C. W. Hulse (1954) in *J. nerv. ment. Dis.*, **119**, 671.

Hill, D. (1948). 'Relationship between Epilepsy and Schizophrenia. E.E.G. Studies.' *Folia psychiat. neurol. neurochir. neerl.*, **51**, 95–111.

Hoagland, H., Bergen, J. R., Koella, W. P. and Freeman, H. (1962). *Ann. N.Y. Acad. Sci.*, **96**, 469.

Ingram, T. T. S. (1965). 'The Neurology of Psychosis in Childhood.' Private Communication to The Working Party on Childhood Schizophrenia (*see* Creak, 1961).

Kallman, F. J. and Roth, B. (1956). 'Genetic Aspects of Pre-adolescent Schizophrenia.' *Am. J. Psychiat.*, **112**, 599–606.

Kaplan, M. (1950). 'An Approach to Psychiatric Problems in Childhood.' *Am. J. Dis. Child.*, **79**, 791–805.

Kay, D. W. K. and Roth, M. (1961). 'Environmental and Hereditary Factors in the Schizophrenias of Old Age (" Late Paraphrenia ") and their Bearing on the General Problem of Causation of Schizophrenia.' *J. ment. Sci.*, **107**, 649–686.

REFERENCES

Klein, M. (1932). *The Psychoanalysis of Children*. London; Hogarth Press.

Klinberg, O. (1935). Negro intelligence and selective migration. New York; *Columiba University Press*.

Koegler, R. R., Colbert, E. G. and Eiduson, S. (1961). 'Wanted: A Biochemical Test for Schizophrenia.' *Calif. Med.*, **94**, 26–29.

Lee, E. S. (1951). Negro intelligence and selective migration. *Amer. Sociol. Rev.* 16, 227.

Mahler, M. S. (1952). 'On Child Psychosis and Schizophrenia: Autistic and Symbiotic Psychosis.' *The Psychoanalytic Study of the Child*, Vol. 7. New York; International Universities Press.

Moncrieff, A. A., Loumides, O. P., Clayton, B. E., Patrick, A. D., Renwick, A. G. C. and Roberts, G. E. (1964). 'Lead Poisoning in Children.' *Archs Dis. Childh.*, **39**, 1.

Norman, E. (1954). 'Reality Relationship in Schizophrenic Children.' *Br. J. med. Psychol.*, **27**, 126.

Nouailhat, F. (1960). 'Schizophrenia in Children. Early Neurological Aspects.' *Fr. méd.*, **23**, 414–415.

O'Gorman, G. (1954). 'Psychosis as a Cause of Mental Defect.' *J. ment. Sci.*, **100**, 934–943.

— (1968). The relationship of severe emotional disorders including psychosis, with intellectual deterioration. International Association for the Scientific Study of Mental Deficiency. (Proceedings of the Montpellier Conference.)

Oliver, B. E. and O'Gorman, G. (1966). 'Blood Lead and Pica in Psychotic Children.' *Develop. Med. Child Neurol.* In Press.

Osmond, H. and Smythies, J. (1952). *J. ment. Sci.*, **98**, 309.

Ounsted, C. (1961). Personal Communication.

Pollin, W., Cardon, P. V. and Ketz, S. S. (1953). *Science*, **204**, 403.

Quastel, J. H. and Quastel, D. M. J. (1962). *The Chemistry of Brain Metabolism in Health and Disease*. Springfield, Ill.; Thomas.

Rabonovitch, R. D., Lucas, A. R., Ingram, W. and Shaw, C. (1965). 'Childhood Schizophrenia: Evolution to Adulthood.' Paper presented to the Annual Meeting of the American Orthopsychiatric Association.

Rimland, B. (1962). *Infantile Autism*. New York; Meredith.

REFERENCES

Rutter, M. (1965). 'The Influence of Organic and Emotional Factors on the Origins, Nature and Outcome of Childhood Psychosis.' *Develop. Med. Child Neurol.*, **7**, 518–28.

Simon, G. B. and Gillies, W. M. (1964). 'Some Physical Characteristics of a Group of Psychotic Children.' *Br. J. Psychiat.*, **110**, 104–107.

Sutton, H. E. and Read, J. H. (1958). 'Abnormal Amino Acid Metabolism in a Case Suggesting Autism.' *A.M.A. J. Dis. Child.*, **96**, 23–28.

Tramer, M. (1935–36). *Z. Kinderpsychiat.*, **1**, 91.

Williams, C. E. (1966). Personal Communication.

Winnicot, D. W. (1953). 'Psychoses and Child Care.' *Br. J. med. Psychol.*, **26**, 68–74.

Yakolev, P., Weinberger, M. and Chipman, C. (1948). 'Heller's Syndrome as a Pattern of Schizophrenic Behaviour Disturbance in Early Childhood.' *Am. J. ment. Def.*, **55**, 318.

Young, J. Z. (1965). In Studies in physiology. Ed: Eccles. Berlin: Springer-Verlag.

INDEX

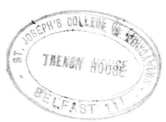